Clinical Audit
and
Epi Info

Antony Stewart

Specialist in Public Health
Rowley Regis & Tipton Primary Care Trust

and

Jammi N Rao

Director of Public Health
North Birmingham Primary Care Trust

Foreword by

Professor Richard Baker

Director
Clinical Governance Research & Development Unit
University of Leicester

Radcliffe Medical Press

Radcliffe Medical Press Ltd
18 Marcham Road
Abingdon
Oxon OX14 1AA
United Kingdom

www.radcliffe-oxford.com
The Radcliffe Medical Press electronic catalogue and online ordering facility.
Direct sales to anywhere in the world.

British Library Cataloguing in Publication Data

A catalogue record for this book is available from the British Library.

ISBN 1 85775 928 1

Typeset by Joshua Associates Ltd, Oxford
Printed and bound by TJ International Ltd, Padstow, Cornwall

Contents

Foreword

Clinical audit is now core business for the NHS and all clinicians who work in it. Audit is critical to the achievement of the type of care that people now expect – timely, based on best current evidence, tailored to their needs and preferences, and delivered in a personal and human way. For more than a decade, clinicians have been encouraged to take part in clinical audit, and been offered training and assistance to make that possible. Many professional groups have made demonstration of the ability to complete successful audit a component of their training programmes, and all NHS trusts have policies to support clinical audit. Such policies include the creation of audit departments, and a key factor in NHS trust audit programmes has been the emergence of a new professional group – the audit support staff who have ensured that the NHS has the skills and local leadership which are so important. Consequently, much progress has been made.

Audit is now practised in various forms: the traditional audit cycle completed on an often annual basis; PDSA (Plan–Do–Study–Act) cycles using small patient samples and sometimes involving rapid cycle data collection; major national audit projects such as MINAP (Myocardial Infarction National Audit Project); reviews of individual cases, as in significant event audit; and projects that involve patients either in providing information about their experiences of care or taking part in standard setting and activities to prompt improvements. With audit as the necessary preliminary step, a comprehensive array of quality improvement systems and structures is being introduced, including, for example, investigation of patterns of adverse events through the National Patient Safety Agency, the correction of poor clinical performance through the National Clinical Assessment Authority, inspection of NHS trusts by the Commission for Health Improvement, and the centrepiece at the local level of clinical governance. Should we now stop to celebrate, to decide that all that we set out to achieve has been accomplished? Perhaps we should spare the time for a short celebration.

Audit and associated quality improvement activities must deliver much more in the coming years. They must contribute to the implementation of National Service Frameworks, guidelines and other guidance issued by the National Institute for Clinical Excellence or SIGN (Scottish Inter-collegiate Guidelines Network), and must help transform clinical services so that they genuinely do meet the expectations of the public. The report of the Bristol Inquiry is just one source of evidence to support this case. Clinicians must now ensure that audit is more successful, more fre-quently, in improving more aspects of care. All too often in the past, audits have not been completed, have not been given the necessary support by managers or healthcare teams, have not taken account of the perspectives of patients and have failed to bring about benefits in patient care. This must change.

Antony Stewart and Jammi Rao's book provides important help in making audit effective as a matter of routine. Their advice on conducting audit is clearly expressed and based on experience, and it will be of value to both clinicians and audit staff. But the technical features of audit can often present difficulties, including the calculation of sample sizes, collec-tion of consistent data and analyses that distinguish the background variations in care from true improvements accounted for by the efforts of healthcare teams. Audit does not, however, need expertise in the use of obscure statistical software. Epi Info is a simple program that solves many of the problems. It is readily available without cost. All it needs is a simple set of instructions on its use in audit. Read on – the following pages contain all you need to know to use Epi Info quickly and efficiently to steer your audits to successful conclusions. Making use of Epi Info with the assistance of this book will help you ensure that your audits do meet the challenges of modern healthcare.

Professor Richard Baker
Director
Clinical Governance Research & Development Unit
University of Leicester
July 2003

Preface

Epi Info is a computer database which *really can* make life easier for you when carrying out clinical audit. It can prove invaluable to GP practices, voluntary organisations, hospital doctors, pharmacists, dentists, clinical audit groups, hospital clinical audit departments and any other organisations that need to collect and analyse data.

Questionnaires and data collection projects can be set up and processed in a matter of minutes, and it makes no difference whether the amount of information you collect is large or small – the program can handle literally billions of records.

Using Epi Info is simple and straightforward. Excellent results can be produced quickly without any experience of computer programming. Another very useful feature of Epi Info is that it costs nothing! Unlimited copies of the program can be made and given to friends and colleagues.

This book is designed to provide you with a reasonable understanding of the principal features of Epi Info v6.04 in a short space of time, so that you can begin using it straight away. Additionally, the fundamentals of clinical audit, clinical governance and medical statistics are discussed and related to Epi Info. Tutorials with working examples and datasets are supplied on a CD-ROM, together with a number of sample clinical audit protocols that you can adapt for your own use.

The full reference manual is accessible from within Epi Info if you require information on the more advanced features available. A further reading list on the topics covered is included at the end of the book.

Clinical audit is an exciting tool which can help bring about real improvements to the care of patients, and Epi Info is a valuable aid to this process. We hope this guide will help you to gain a basic under-standing of clinical audit and Epi Info, and encourage you to make regular use of them both.

Antony Stewart
Jammi N Rao
July 2003

Acknowledgements

Portions of this book were previously published by Brixton Books, and we are grateful to Tracey Greenwood and Mark Myatt for allowing their publication here.

Dedications

AS – Books take countless hours to write, and this has been stolen from time that should be spent with the people I cherish most. So I thank my family Jenny, Katie, Michael and my mother Edith for understanding my frequent absences from their lives.

But my share of this book is dedicated to Olive Parker, who also has always believed in me, giving unlimited time, encouragement and love. You are and always have been a wonderful Aunt – thank you!

You all have my deepest love.

JNR – To my mum who appreciated books despite not having had a formal education herself; and to my dad who taught me to appreciate maths.

I am also deeply grateful to my wife, Vidya, a busy paediatrician, and to my sons Vikram, Gopal and Venkat, for all their encouragement and support.

1

Clinical governance

Clinical governance and the central role of clinical audit

Clinical governance is the programme of work through which the NHS is committed to improving clinical quality. The initiative was launched in 1998 as part of a major reform of the health service following Labour's return to power in 1997. Its purpose was 'to ensure that clinical standards are met, and that processes are in place to ensure continuous improvement in quality' (Department of Health, 1998). For the first time a statutory duty was proposed for trusts concerned with the quality of their services. The chief executive was to be charged not only with the responsibility of ensuring that there was continuous improvement in clinical quality, but also with the duty to report to the board on the state of clinical quality. Trusts were to be given a new statutory duty for the quality of clinical services. Unlike the clinical audit programme that preceded it, clinical quality was no longer solely a professional responsibility that managers could leave to clinicians.

Clinical governance was defined as 'a system through which NHS organisations are accountable for continuously improving the quality of their services and safeguarding high standards of care by creating an environment in which excellence in clinical care will flourish' – a definition accredited to the Chief Medical Officer, Sir Liam Donaldson.

The components of clinical governance

- Evidence-based medicine
- Lifelong learning and continuous professional development
- Needs assessment
- Clinical audit
- National standards (laid down by bodies such as the National Institute for Clinical Excellence and monitored by the Commission for Health Audit and Improvement)
- Risk management
- Patient involvement

The role of clinical audit as a component of clinical governance

There was widespread interest in, and also welcome for, the proposals. There were some who felt that, with its emphasis on all the many other functions listed in the box (above), the days of clinical audit were numbered. Clinical governance was felt to have superseded clinical audit, which itself had been introduced earlier in 1991 as part of the internal market reforms of the NHS.

However, those in the business of clinical quality were in no doubt that the clinical governance initiative, far from abolishing the need for robust clinical audit, actually strengthened the need for it. By placing clinical quality at the centre of the new agenda for managers, clinical governance made it all the more imperative that there was continual, timely and valid measurement of quality – and that is what clinical audit is really about.

The key to understanding why clinical audit is in fact at the heart of clinical governance is to go back to the definition of clinical governance and to appreciate the words 'continuous improvements in quality'. Clinical governance is thus not about where you are with respect to quality, but which direction you are moving in. The continuous nature of the process is best described in the PDSA cycle – a standard quality improvement tool used in the best clinical units (Berwick, 1996).

The PDSA cycle

Model for improvement

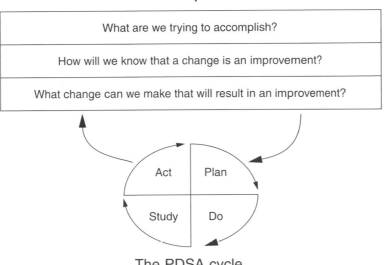

The PDSA cycle.
(Source: Langley *et al.*, 1992)

PDSA stands for **Plan–Do–Study–Act**. The first stage is to Plan one or more series of actions that will be implemented with a clearly defined objective in mind. Ideally it should involve a critical review of the relevant research literature; this ensures that the steps that are proposed are more rather than less likely to result in a beneficial outcome. The second stage is to implement these proposals. This is the 'Do' phase. Invariably, implementation is incomplete. Not all members of the team may be signed up to the change; the methods by which the change is put in place may result in partial uptake; and the team members may slip back into the old way of doing things (see 'Introducing change', p. 24). It is the job of those who manage the service to make sure that the plan is implemented, however incompletely.

The third phase is to Study some aspect of the system to see whether the desired change has been achieved. Are people getting their thrombolysis within the stated time-limits? Are all people with diabetes having their eye tests done? Is their blood pressure being measured?

The results of the Study should lead directly to action to change the system in some way in order further to enhance the quality. If the desired effects are not seen at all, then it may be time to question the original planned change and scrap it altogether. If some members of the team are not adopting the changed way of working then the action might be to investigate why.

The Plan, the Do and the Act phases of the PDSA cycle are for clinicians and managers to work on. The Study phase is fundamentally what clinical audit is all about. If it is well designed and rigorously carried out, intelligently analysed and clearly presented, clinical audit, used as part of the PDSA cycle, can be a powerful lever for the 'continuous improvement in clinical quality' that is clinical governance.

2

Clinical audit

What is clinical audit?

Clinical audit is all about improving the care that patients receive. It is essentially just a process of self-evaluation – a way of improving patient care and your practice by looking at what you do, then establishing whether you can do it better. It is defined as 'the systematic and critical analysis of the quality of clinical care, including the procedures used for the diagnosis, treatment and care, the associated use of resources and the resulting outcome and quality of life for the patient' (NHS Executive, 1996).

Clinical audit is 'an important tool for determining whether actual performance compares with evidence-based standards and, if not, what changes are needed to improve performance' (Chambers and Boath, 2000). Contrary to popular belief, clinical audit does not have to be a complicated and laborious process. It is often most effective when kept simple – then it is easy and not very time-consuming. When done well, audit is a rewarding exercise which can yield valuable results. It is worth noting that audit projects which fail usually do so because of bad planning and execution.

Audit can bring many benefits which can help you as well as your patients:

- **Improved patient care and satisfaction**. The main aim of audit.
- **Education**. As you carry out audit, you learn more about the topic concerned and how things may be improved.
- **Better teamworking**. You do not need to do audit alone: it is easier when everyone is involved, and your team will work better when you all have a common purpose. The National Institute for Clinical Excellence (NICE, 2002) states that 'Clinical audit projects are best

conducted within a structured programme, with effective leadership, participation by all staff, and an emphasis on team working and support.'

- **More effective communication**. Specific audits can evaluate communication systems and improve them. Also, teams working on an audit will almost certainly find their lines of communication improved by the processes of co-operating and learning to find out what is going on, and suggesting ways of improvement.
- **Providing hard evidence to justify changes**. The results produced by well-executed audit provide hard evidence of what is actually happening. So long as the methods of data collection and analysis are sound, audit can be a powerful tool that is hard to ignore.
- **Enhanced quality of working life**. You can use audit to help change bad working practices, which will benefit your working life as well as patient care.
- **Increased efficiency**. Audit can identify inefficient systems and help get them changed.
- **Maximised funding or income for your organisation**. Hard evidence produced by audit can be invaluable in securing funding for particular projects. For example, in primary care audit can be used to ensure that all payments (such as those for immunisation targets, contraceptive advice, etc.) can be and are being claimed.

Although a great deal has been written about audit, it is essentially very easy. A set of six steps, called the audit cycle, have been developed to make things more straightforward.

The audit cycle made easy

Doing audit is simple – just follow the six easy steps around the audit cycle:

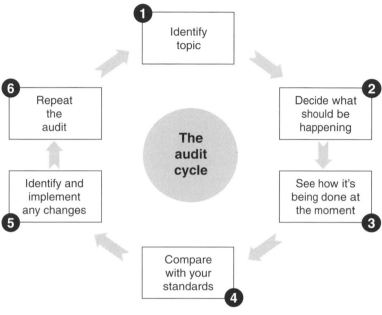

The audit cycle.

Step 1. Identify your topic

This can be an area of concern, a current problem or just something that interests you. For example, how long your patients are having to wait before being seen at the surgery or clinic, whether regular eye checks are being arranged for patients with diabetes, or taking a look at prescribing for a particular condition. Remember that your topic can be organisational as well as clinical, so anyone (or everyone) can be involved.

Step 2. Decide what should be happening

Think about how you would really like to see things happening with regard to your topic. Then decide how often you want to see it actually taking place (e.g. 90% of the time). By doing this, you are setting criteria and standards. Try to ensure that your criteria and standards are realistic and are clinically proven where appropriate. In the following example:

- 90% of patients who are identified as being hypertensive should have had their blood pressure measured within the last 12 months

'90%' is the *standard*; the rest is the *criteria*.

Step 3. See how it's being done now

This involves observing what is actually happening and collecting data to measure it over a specified period of time. It can be quite a surprise to see what really is going on when you look hard. Although this exercise may sound time-consuming, it need not take long at all. Good planning, well-designed data collection forms and the involvement of other practice team members can make the task significantly lighter. At the end of the period the information you have collected can be analysed and will then give a picture of what is actually going on.

Step 4. Compare with original standards

See if there is any difference between the standards you originally set up at step 2 and the results you have obtained at step 3.

Step 5. Identify and implement any changes

If your standards and your results differ, it is useful to identify why this is so. If you know the reasons why particular areas are not performing as well as you would wish, you can make changes and improve standards. You may find that the data collection and subsequent analysis show that your standards *are* being met. In this case, the audit will still have been useful for your peace of mind and for proving how well you are doing.

Step 6. Repeat the audit

It is *essential* to repeat the audit after, say, six months or a year. This will indicate how effective any changes have been, or whether you should review the situation further. This process of evaluation and change can make tangible improvements to the way you work.

The audit protocol

Before starting an audit, it makes sense to plan everything carefully. It is also advisable to produce an **audit protocol** – a document detailing the aims of the audit, criteria and standards, how it will be carried out and how the results will be actioned. Examples of audit protocols are shown in Chapters 5 and 10.

What can be audited – and in what ways?

You can audit just about any aspect of activity – from how many patients have to wait in outpatients, to the appropriateness of antibiotic prescribing. If it affects how you do things, and can be measured, it can be audited. Avedis Donabedian (1966) categorised healthcare quality under three main headings.

Structure

These audits are concerned with the resources that facilitate the process of care. Examples of structure audits include:

* number of patients on a particular list
* facilities available for patient care
* patient satisfaction with waiting room facilities
* ratio of patients to nurses.

Process

These are concerned with the activities of those involved in the care of patients. Examples of process audits include:

* items recorded in patients' notes
* tests carried out
* types and quantities of drugs prescribed
* numbers of consultations.

Outcome

These are concerned with the **results** of healthcare. They can be viewed as the product of structures and processes. Outcome audits are popular because they show directly how the care of patients has been affected. An audit which shows that adequate facilities are available, or that better referral letters are being sent by GPs to consultants, implies that better care will result. An outcome audit showing that certain interventions have reduced postoperative infection rates demonstrates that a positive outcome to patient care has resulted.

Examples of outcome audits include:

- the incidence of teenage pregnancies following a campaign promoting emergency contraception
- the number of days off work/school taken by patients following an audit evaluating the appropriateness of asthma management
- the proportion of patients without coronary heart disease (CHD) who smoke, and have received smoking cessation advice.

Audits can be **prospective** (where data collection begins after a specified date) or **retrospective** (where data are extracted from existing records).

A vast array of topics can be used for audit, but subjects highlighted by National Service Frameworks (NSFs) as well as national and local priorities will be especially suitable.

Clinical guidelines

Clinical guidelines are designed to aid clinicians in the diagnosis and management of certain clinical conditions by providing a recommended set of instructions on what should be done and how it should be carried out. These guidelines often contain auditable standards, so that the effectiveness of the guideline, and hence the resulting quality of patient care, can be assessed.

Clinically effective practice

The best audits are those which are based on clinically effective practice. This can be defined as 'the extent to which specific clinical interventions, when deployed in the field for a particular patient or population, do what they are intended to do, i.e. maintain and improve health and secure the greatest possible health gain from the available resources' (NHS Executive, 1996). It involves 'the use of current best evidence in the care of individual patients' (van Zwanenberg and Harrison, 2000).

In clinical audit, this means that the criteria and standards are based on practice which has been well researched and proven to be effective (also known as evidence-based medicine). For example, there is evidence that low-dose aspirin should be prescribed or advised for patients with angina, unless contraindicated (Antiplatelet Trialists' Collaboration, 1994).

An audit based on clinically effective practice could therefore entail identifying every patient with angina, and checking whether they are being given or advised to take aspirin therapy. Those who are not, could be started on aspirin immediately, unless contraindicated. A clear outcome of better patient care is likely to result.

Audit and research

Audit is not the same as research. Research projects – clinical trials, retrospective studies, prospective epidemiological studies and surveys – are carried out to answer specific questions. Clinical audit is an essential and principal component of a programme of clinical quality improvement. It is central to the implementation of clinically effective practice that previous research studies have shown to be effective.

The NICE defines audit as:

Clinical audit is a quality improvement process that seeks to improve patient care and outcomes through systematic review of care against explicit criteria and the implementation of change. Aspects of the structure, processes and outcomes of care are selected and systematically evaluated against explicit criteria. Where indicated, changes are implemented at an individual, team or service level and further monitoring is used to confirm improvement in health-care delivery.
(NICE, 2003)

Research is much wider and seeks to answer more fundamental questions. In the clinical context, both research and audit have to do with the processes of clinical care. Research asks and addresses the questions: 'What processes of care will yield better outcomes?' and 'Does this treatment work?' Clinical audit answers the question: 'Are we carrying out the care processes that we set out to deliver?'

Two questions often arise: 'How methodologically rigorous must my audit project be?' and 'Do I need permission from an ethics committee?'

Methodological rigour

Although audit and research are different, they both need equal methodological rigour in planning, case selection, data collection and analysis, and interpretation. It is a common misconception that these principles apply only to research studies. It is true that researchers would like to be able to generalise their results to a wider population of subjects. This quest for generalisability leads to an insistence on good design and careful planning and execution of the study. However, the results of a clinical audit project, if they are to be of any value at all, also need to be valid, reproducible and generalisable to all the patients who will be cared for in that clinical unit. If they are not, then it is unlikely that the results of audit will lead to changes in the way care is delivered. Good design – including sampling procedure and minimisation of bias – reliable recording of data and appropriate and technically accurate analysis are therefore no less important.

Ethics committee approval

Clinical audit often requires the collection of patient-related clinical data. 'Does this need ethics committee approval?' is a question that both clinicians and audit staff often ask. There is uncertainty in many peoples' minds; unfortunately, there is not an agreed set of criteria that would allow an unambiguous judgement in each and every case. General principles can be laid down to guide a decision.

The Central Office for Research Ethics Committees (COREC) requires that researchers seek ethics committee approval for research studies that involve:

- NHS patients, i.e. those subjects recruited by virtue of their past or present treatment by the NHS, including those treated under contract with the private sector.
- Foetal material and *in vitro* fertilisation involving NHS patients.
- The recently dead in NHS premises.
- Access to records of past and present NHS patients.
- The use of, or potential access to, NHS premises or facilities (including NHS staff).

(Central Office for Research Ethics Committees, 2003)

Clinical audit does often involve the use of patient data and so the confusion is understandable. The most logical position to take is to consider any project as research unless it satisfies each of the following criteria:

1 The proposed study involves collecting and analysing patient data that do not require any extension of current routine clinical practice. (If there is to be a departure from routine clinical processes for the sake of the project then it is not a simple audit.)
2 There is no possibility that patient-related data will be stored, transmitted or analysed outside the healthcare organisation where the care takes place.

3 There is no involvement of staff who are not directly involved in the patients' care or staff who are not employed by the healthcare organisation.
4 The results of the clinical audit are solely for the purpose of quality improvement and therefore there is no intention formally to publish the findings beyond the healthcare organisation.

Audit by nature is a critical examination of one's own practice. Therefore projects initiated by third parties and that set out to answer questions such as 'How well do GPs treat hypertension?', and invite practices to collect and pass on data to a central database are clearly research.

By these criteria, multicentre registers of patients with a defined diagnosis, collaborative audit projects such as those conducted by medical royal colleges or prospective databanks funded and run by commercial sponsors are not simple clinical audits; they are clearly research, and it is best to seek formal ethics committee approval.

The obvious distinction in practical terms is that research – even if it only involves data collection and analysis – needs formal explicit patient consent. Clinical audit, on the other hand, does not expose the patients involved to any risk of potential breach of confidentiality, and so does not call for explicit consent.

There will always be situations when it is not easy to be certain whether or not ethics committee permission is appropriate. In such circumstances it is best to err on the side of caution and apply to the relevant research ethics committee (see www.corec.org.uk for details of your nearest research ethics committee).

Patient satisfaction audit and questionnaire design

Some survey style audits, such as those based on patient satisfaction, can be useful so long as they contain explicit criteria and standards and have the potential to make improvements (e.g. 80% of patients should say they are satisfied with the surgery's repeat prescription service).

When planning a **questionnaire**-based audit, remember to keep the forms as short and simple as possible, preferably no more than one or two sides of A4 paper. If the questionnaire is too long or complicated, fewer patients will take the trouble to complete it. Ask your questions clearly, so they cannot be misunderstood (e.g. a question of 'Are you male or female?' will usually generate at least one answer of 'Yes').

Avoid **leading** questions or your results will be inaccurate and you will lose credibility when the results are published (e.g. 'Do you agree that our clinic provides an excellent service?'). Start the questionnaire with an explanation of why you are doing it and how respondents can help you (and themselves) if they fill it in.

The first question should interest the respondent enough to *want* to answer it. People often react well to the fact that you are taking an interest in them, so it is usually advisable to begin by asking about things like their age, gender and occupation.

Try to use questions giving a range of choices:

- **Yes/No**
  Do you feel that the physiotherapist spent enough time with you? *(tick one box)*
  ☐ Yes   ☐ No
- **A selection of answers**
  How long did you have to wait in the clinic before being seen by the physiotherapist? *(tick one box)*
  Less than 10 minutes ☐
  Between 10 minutes and half an hour ☐
  Over half an hour ☐
- **Likert scales**. The Likert scale is a method of answering a question by selecting one of a range of numbers (e.g. 1 = excellent; 2 = good; 3 = fair; 4 = bad; 5 = very bad) in preference to open questions which can yield large amounts of text that is difficult to analyse.
  How do you rate the overall service you received at the physiotherapy clinic? *(tick one box)*
  1 Excellent ☐   2 Good ☐   3 Fair ☐   4 Bad ☐   5 Very bad ☐

Likert-scale questions can have either an even or an odd number of responses. Using an odd number gives respondents the chance to opt for the middle ground (e.g. a choice of excellent/good/fair/bad/very bad allows them to say they are neither happy nor unhappy by choosing 'fair'). Using an even number avoids this, forcing them to go either one way or the other. It is up to you to decide which is best for your particular situation.

It is good practice to stress confidentiality and not to ask for name and address data, as some patients will avoid making negative comments for fear of jeopardising their future treatment.

Be aware that a postal questionnaire might achieve a response rate of only around 25%. It is better to ask people to complete the form and hand it in before they leave you if possible (they may find it easier if you provide a pen), or be prepared to send a number of reminders. Sending reminders will be easier if you have remembered to use an identity code on the original questionnaire so that you know exactly who has failed to respond though doing this will, of course, hinder anonymity. Enclosing a stamped addressed envelope (SAE) with a postal questionnaire may improve response rates.

Finally, remember that satisfaction questionnaires are sometimes regarded as 'happy sheets'. Respondents tend to err on the side of happiness, possibly because they don't want to upset anyone or they are scared of getting poor treatment the next time they see you. Phrase your questions with this in mind if you want to maximise your chances of securing accurate and honest answers.

Significant event audit

Another type of audit to consider is significant event audit. This usually involves the retrospective examination of a single major event which has resulted in an unsatisfactory outcome. Examples of such events include:

- late diagnosis of cancer
- suicide
- leaking of sensitive information.

Initially, two questions should be asked:

- Could anything have been done to prevent this event from happening?
- Can anything now be done to prevent it from happening again?

Correcting any problems or deficiencies discovered during the course of the audit can lead to better patient care and provide benefits to the whole practice team. Factors such as efficiency, understanding working relationships and motivation can be enhanced when this audit method is used correctly. It is, of course, very important to choose a suitable event, as a good result will only be achieved if there is scope for real improvement.

In each case, a systematic examination should take place to establish the following:

- The circumstances of the incident.
- Relevant history from patient notes, staff recollections, etc.
- Whether anything could reasonably have been done to prevent it.
- What lessons can be learned to avoid future occurrences.
- What action should now be taken.

At first, significant event auditing may sound quite daunting, owing to the fear that a particular person's mistakes or shortcomings might be exposed during the investigation. However, significant event auditing can be one of the most productive and effective forms of clinical audit. It should, however, be remembered that one of the fundamental reasons for doing audit is to learn from experiences and mistakes, so that improvements can be made. The aim is to ensure high standards while reducing the possibility of errors in the future, and not to place the blame on someone unless it is absolutely necessary to do so.

It is difficult to ensure complete confidentiality, but this can be achieved if care and sensitivity are used. This method of auditing can be undertaken by an individual practice member, so no one else need know anything about the investigation. However, more effective results will be obtained if all or part of the practice team work together on the audit to agreed and established rules of confidentiality, adopting a 'no-blame' approach. If all enquiries are handled sensitively, with a clear understanding that the intention is to secure improvements rather than apportion individual blame, no one need feel threatened.

Focus groups

Focus groups are a research tool which can be useful for obtaining large amounts of information very quickly. This makes them suitable for the data collection stage of certain audits. For example, a patient satisfaction audit using a questionnaire may tell you that your patients are satisfied with your overall service, but the use of focus groups will help you to find out more detailed information about what they are happy with, and what they are not. In other words, focus groups allow you to delve deeper into how people feel.

They normally take the form of several small groups, each answering a number of standardised questions on a given topic. The answers that the groups (and their individual members) give will provide the information. These groups can be useful for:

- planning health services
- evaluating health needs
- providing information to help decision making.

They are less useful for:

- involving local users or the general public in decision making
- informing local people about changes in services
- establishing local service priorities.

Three or more groups should be used, each containing around eight participants. The participants in each group should have similar characteristics. This means that the people in each group are classified by some means (e.g. age, social class, ethnic origin, clinical specialities, chronic disease, etc.). The nature of the classification should be chosen to be appropriate for the subject to be discussed. For example, the age classification may be most useful if the groups are focusing on care of the elderly, and ethnic origin may be best for the subject of providing services for local ethnic minority groups. The more groups you use, the better feel you will get for the issue concerned. A common method of determining the number of groups required is **sampling to redundancy.** Under this scheme you continue to convene focus groups until no new information is revealed.

Group participants need to be carefully selected according to the classifications you have decided for the groups concerned. Choose the meeting venue carefully, too. Will it be accessible for everyone? Will there be enough space for everyone you need to accommodate? Always provide refreshments and, if possible, reimburse travel expenses. Let the participants know about this when you invite them.

Construct a list of questions which all the groups will be asked, and consider them carefully. The format of a focus group meeting will normally be:

- Introduction.
- A general question to break the ice among participants.
- Questions, moving from general to specific, and from easy to difficult, or even threatening.

A word of warning here – these groups need someone with good facilitation skills if they are to be successful. This means that the person facilitating should have:

- experience of arranging and conducting focus groups
- knowledge of the stages involved
- understanding of group dynamics.

It is therefore a good idea to either acquire these skills for yourself before embarking on a focus group, or get a skilled person to facilitate for you. It helps if someone can take notes at the meetings (not the facilitator, who will be busy doing other things). Use a good-quality tape recorder with a conference microphone to make a back-up of the proceedings.

Analysing the content of the meetings also requires skill, time and patience. Remember that the data produced will be mainly **qualitative**. Therefore think very carefully about how you will analyse the data, and do so in a systematic way.

Where will I find the time to do audit?

You may well agree that audit is a worthwhile activity, but as a busy professional where will you find the time to do it? Fortunately, audit does not have to be complicated and time-consuming. Some of the most effective audits are short, simple and well focused. Certainly audit will take up some of your time, but this can be minimised by the following.

- Involve other members of your team in the audit – many hands make light work.
- Concentrate your audits on small areas of activity – for example, you can't audit the whole spectrum of diabetes in a single audit, so why not just examine one aspect now and look at another aspect later (e.g. how many patients over 40 years of age with diabetes have had their feet examined in the past 18 months?).
- Spend a little time thinking carefully about how the audit should be carried out. Make sure that everyone involved knows what is expected of them.
- Ask your local organisations (e.g. primary care trust) for help. Audit grants may be available to pay for staff overtime or materials.
- Tackle the audit in stages – there's no need to do it all at once.
- Remember that audit has the potential to make real improvements. That is worth spending some time on!
- Finally, some audits can *save* you time by increasing efficiency, thereby reducing wastage. Why not plan an audit with this in mind?

The skills required to do audit are transferable to research and communicable disease control. It is a good idea to build data collection, management and analysis skills on audit before graduating to research. If possible, try to set aside a little time each week for audit.

When done properly you will find audit a most rewarding and useful activity.

Getting help with audit in the UK

If you work in primary care your local primary care trust may be able to help. If you are in secondary or tertiary care your local trust may have a clinical audit department. Some primary care audit groups have changed their name to reflect the principal focus of the work, and most primary care trusts have their own clinical audit staff. You should be able to find assistance with all aspects of audit, including:

- **Planning the audit**. What to audit, and the best way to go about it.
- **Data collection**. The most effective methods to achieve the purpose.
- **Data analysis**. Producing results from the information you collect.
- **Presentation of results**. The best methods of getting the message across.
- **Implementing change**. How to ensure the audit results in improvements.
- **Helping with literature searches**. Making your audit more credible by providing evidence of research which supports your criteria and standards.

Audit groups normally offer one-to-one support with audit if required, or even just occasional advice. However, they will not do the whole of the audit for you. Audit is an educational activity and you will learn a lot from the experience of working through a well-designed audit project. Audit groups often organise training courses, which are sometimes accredited by professional bodies.

Some private sector organisations provide all or some of the services listed above.

Twelve golden rules for successful audit

Well-planned audits should be relatively easy to carry out and will enhance your practice and help your patients. Badly planned audits will just waste resources. Whenever you plan an audit, however simple, it makes sense to spend a little time to consider whether you are following these rules.

1 **Make sure that your chosen topic interests you**
   It will be difficult to sustain enthusiasm for an audit that does not inspire you. Teams selecting an audit topic should ensure that all, or most, of its members are interested in doing an audit on that particular subject. But remember that boring topics can still be very important for patient care.

2 **Start with topics where you suspect there is a need for change**
   There will always be a place for audits that are carried out just to check whether areas of practice come up to scratch. It is a good idea, for example, to consider starting with a subject where you think something may be going wrong. Topics centred around national targets or local priorities may also provide a trigger for you to start an audit.

   Audits that quickly result in tangible improvements in patient care will motivate you and your team to continue auditing. Be careful to avoid audits that employ unethical methodologies (e.g. putting patients at any kind of risk or pressurising them into participating or revealing their identities) or consider conditions that are seen too rarely to be audited effectively. Note that rare conditions are good subjects for significant event audits.

3 **Don't go it alone**

Ideally, several people should be involved. Audit is much simpler if you involve your colleagues at every stage. Not only will this drastically lighten the workload, but you will probably encounter less resistance when it comes to making changes to current practices.

4 **Keep it short and simple**

Try to audit small areas of activity at a time. Many projects are abandoned at an early stage because of over-ambitious plans which prove impossible to carry out in the time available. For the same reason, avoid carrying out audits over extended periods. Beware of extremes: collect data over too short a time and your audit will be unreliable; over too long a time and you and your staff and patients will be likely to tire of the project and give up, resulting in wasted effort and frustration. Most simple projects will yield reliable results when data collection lasts between one and four weeks, but this depends on the sample size used (*see* Chapter 8). Always set a timescale for your audit, and make every effort to keep to it.

5 **Use realistic criteria and standards**

Don't set your standards so high that they are unattainable, or so low that they fail to represent good clinical practice. The standard you set should be the minimum standard that you consider acceptable. Of course, some standards will always need to be 100% (e.g. all patients to be given aspirin following myocardial infarction unless contra-indicated), while others would arguably be acceptable with a standard of 70% (e.g. patients should be seen within 15 minutes of their appointment time).

Strive for excellence by all means, but remember that we all work in the real world. Your criteria and standards will be more credible if they are backed up with research evidence which proves them to be effective. Make an effort to find out if any such evidence exists (*see* Chapter 3).

Your local clinical audit department or medical library should be able to help you by carrying out a literature search to find any relevant literature. Additionally, your medical library may well have access to computer-based CD-ROM or Internet search systems such as MEDLINE. These allow you to search quickly and effortlessly through an enormous amount of literature to find references (and often brief summaries) on literature that contains information on your chosen subject. The library can then use these references to locate the literature or order a hard copy of the full document for you. 'On-line' services such as MEDLINE are also available via the Internet. *See* Chapter 3 for more information on searching for evidence.

6 **Think it through**

Plan a strategy for carrying out the audit. Consider carefully how you are going to work through all the stages of the audit cycle before proceeding. It will be helpful to prepare an audit protocol detailing the aims of the audit, criteria and standards, how it will be carried out and how the results will be actioned. There are some example audit protocols later in this book (*see* Chapters 5 and 10).

Try to anticipate any possible difficulties that may prevent the audit from succeeding. For example, if your audit is likely to result in improvements involving extra financial costs, will you be able to meet these? If not, consider whether it is worthwhile to proceed with that particular audit.

7 **Think data collection**

Don't collect more data than you actually need. By the same token, avoid collecting so little data that you cannot draw any useful conclusions. Produce data collection forms to record information in a clear and methodical way. Consider how you will analyse the data. On patient questionnaires, for example, it is easier to analyse the answers to 'Yes/No', 'Selection of answers' or 'Likert scale' questions than long, open questions. Make sure that everyone involved in the project understands exactly what they should be doing. Always keep in mind the questions you require answers to and settle for asking just enough. It is often a good idea to make a draft of the tables and reports that you would like the audit to produce. This will allow you to work backwards towards the data you need to collect.

You should strike a balance between sample sizes that are too small, which will yield data that are unreliable, and very large samples, which will be onerous to collect. Aim for the largest sample that you can comfortably and realistically collect within the audit period (*see* Chapter 8).

When carrying out an audit, you cannot always collect data from *all* of the patients concerned. For example, conducting a patient satisfaction audit on all of your patients would probably involve asking several thousand people over a period of several years. If, on the other hand, you were to ask only a few, you risk accidentally selecting all of the patients who have complained about you, or you may even decide to cheat by asking only those who have sent letters of praise.

You can compromise by sending questionnaires to a randomly selected sample of people that is large enough to yield an answer which is likely to be as accurate as if you had asked every patient (e.g. if you wish to ask one-third of your diabetic patients, you could use

systematic sampling. Obtain an alphabetical list of their names and methodically select every third name – by doing this, the list is doing the selecting instead of you). Methods of sampling and sample size calculation are discussed at greater length in Chapter 8. Look at the list carefully before you start selecting. For example, every tenth patient on a list of married people will result in every person being male or every person being female (Donaldson and Donaldson, 2000).

8 **Pilot the audit**

Carry out a short 'dry run' of the audit before launching into the real thing. This will allow you to identify and correct any errors in your audit methodology. The pilot need not take long, and could save you hours of wasted effort. It is worth piloting the questionnaire on your colleagues or a small sample of your study population before committing to a full-scale study.

9 **Analyse the data**

This may seem obvious, but people sometimes collect their data then hide them away, never to be seen again. See the project through. Ask for help with data analysis if necessary (*see* Chapter 7). Only by examining the data properly can you evaluate your performance.

10 **Implement change**

The purpose of audit is to improve patient care. If your audit shows that all of your standards have been met, ask yourself whether they might have been set too low. If you are convinced that the standards were correctly set, then congratulate yourself. You have proved what a good service you give. If you have not met your standards, congratulate yourself anyway. You now know that something is wrong, and have the chance to put it right. If you correct any problems effectively, you have improved the care of your patients. Turn to p. 24 for methods of introducing change.

11 **Share your results, and don't blame anyone**

Adopt a 'no-blame' approach. If your audit highlights a deficiency of any kind, use this as a learning experience and make every effort to put it right. If you have conducted an audit involving patient opinion, post the results on the surgery or clinic wall so that your patients know their efforts were put to good use. Tell them what you have done in response to the details they have provided. If this is not appropriate, make any interested parties aware of your findings.

Even if the results are not good, this at least shows that you are monitoring your practice. Furthermore, by describing how you need to correct any problems, your audit will have improved patient care and you will be a winner. Of course, you may feel that you cannot share your results with others. If so, do not be despondent – just make the improvements and be happy in the knowledge that your time has been well spent.

12 **Repeat the audit**

After a certain amount of time has elapsed (six months or a year), repeat the audit using the same methodology to ensure compatibility between the two audits. This will indicate how effective any changes have been or whether you should review the situation further. The audit should be easier this time, because you will already have done all the planning and have more experience of auditing. Running the same audit regularly provides constant monitoring of what is happening.

Fears, confidentiality and blame

At first, many individuals are scared of audit, expecting it to be a formal investigation which is likely to bring blame and criticism raining down upon them. But audit exists to produce improvements and education – not blame. If anything is discovered to be wrong during an audit project, it should be used as an educational exercise from which all will hopefully learn. This is known as the **no-blame approach**, and helps make audit a positive process.

Confidentiality is another area of concern. People often worry that sensitive information or patients' personal details may be revealed as a result of audit. It is fairly easy to guarantee complete confidentiality by the use of coding systems or anonymity. So long as the 'no-blame' approach is made known and guarantees of anonymity explicitly stated, resistance to audit will be greatly reduced.

Interfacing primary and secondary care audit

It is becoming widely recognised that the care of patients does not always stay within just one area of healthcare. For instance, a patient may consult a GP, be referred to a hospital consultant, undergo surgery and spend some time in the care of a community nurse. This patient has thus come into contact with primary, secondary and tertiary care in a single healthcare episode. Audit projects should be able to follow this care through all of its stages. When an audit follows patients or processes through more than one healthcare agency, it is known as an **interface audit**. This type of audit benefits patients because it monitors the whole of their care, rather than just one part of it. Also, patients tend not to appreciate the thresholds between agencies, seeing their care as one seamless process anyway.

This is much more likely to identify problems, many of which are at the interface of the care agencies (e.g. delays in GP referral letters reaching hospital consultants). Interface audit can also benefit the agencies themselves, because it encourages better communication, problem solving and efficiency.

For this method of audit to work well, the agencies involved should agree on the audit methodology and adopt a 'no-blame' approach. Both will hopefully benefit from the audit, and patient care should be improved as a result. Blaming each other for mistakes will not benefit patients. Improvements will only result from education and the implementation of change. Explicit agreement should be reached on who will do what, and by when, to ensure the smooth running of the exercise.

Examples of interface audit topics include:

- aspects of leg ulcer management in primary, secondary and tertiary care
- appropriateness of GP referrals to orthopaedic surgeons for lower back pain
- quality of hospital discharge letters sent to GPs
- care given to women who present with a breast lump.

Although single-agency audits will always be valuable, audits which interface between agencies can give a better indication of patient care and are more likely to have their recommendations acted upon because each side will have a sense of 'ownership' of the audit. Note that interface audits may become bogged down in bureaucracy and institutional in-fighting unless they are carefully and firmly controlled.

Introducing change

Introducing changes as a result of audit can sometimes be difficult because of opposition from groups and individuals. How many times have we heard people protesting about a forthcoming change, saying '. . . but we've always done it like this, and it's worked alright up to now . . .'? Resistance to change will always be hard to overcome, and at the outset may seem impossible. People tend to be afraid of the unknown, and should be treated with sensitivity and understanding when established working methods need to be changed. Managers who understand why people resist change may be better able to deal with it constructively (NHS Centre for Reviews, University of York, 1999).

The fact is that change can be a destabilising process, and to implement change effectively we need to understand how the world around us works, and be able to predict the outcomes of different courses of action (Upton and Brooks, 1995). Making improvements always requires a degree of change, and improving healthcare quality involves changing the way things are done (Garside, 1998).

It is possible that you will experience no resistance at all to any planned changes. On the other hand, you may encounter huge problems. If the latter happens, you may want to consider using one or more of the following methods:

- Japanese Kaizen theory says: 'If you cannot change, you cannot improve'. Change is no good for its own sake, but audit is a method of making things better than they are now. Improvements resulting from good audit will benefit everyone, making the pain of having to change worthwhile. Keep telling this to people who oppose you.
- If you involve other people in your audit from the outset, they are likely to support any changes because they have a vested interest in the matter.
- Lobby individuals in private and try to win them over to your cause. This will allow you to present a well-argued case and discuss it rationally. It is often easier than persuading whole groups, whose strength is in their numbers.
- If an individual (rather than a group) is opposing you, use the above method to get the majority on your side, one by one.
- Make great efforts to educate and communicate well with all concerned.
- Just do it! This option can be tricky but sometimes works. If the change only involves your own working practices, it is sometimes easier and more effective to simply make the changes and carry on. Consider local circumstances though – at one extreme you may be credited as a superb user of initiative; at the other, you could be branded as a renegade troublemaker.

Some of the following change management theories may be helpful.

Force field analysis (Lewin, 1951)

This assumes that two sets of forces are at work, in any change situation:

1 those driving the change
2 those opposing or restraining it.

If driving forces are *stronger* than opposing forces, progress will be made. This is illustrated in the following diagram, where thicker arrows represent stronger forces:

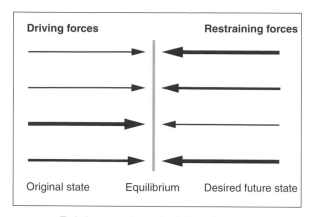

Driving and restraining forces.

It can be useful to cluster forces under specific headings (e.g. personal, interpersonal, inter-group, organisational, technological, environmental). After producing a diagram for your situation, consider what can be done to reduce opposing forces. No attempts should be made to strengthen the driving forces, however. Force field analysis gives a realistic picture of the forces in play.

Commitment planning

A chart is drawn up, showing key personnel, their individual levels of both current and required commitment:

- Not committed – likely to oppose change.
- Let – will not oppose or actively support.
- Help – will support, if someone else leads.
- Make – will lead change and make it happen.

An example chart is illustrated below:

Key players	Not committed	Let	Help	Make
Chief executive	o	————————>		X
Nurse manager			o X	
PCG chair		o ————————>		X
PH consultant	o ————————>	X		
Social worker		o —> X		
GP			X <— o	
Facilitator				o X
Health Visitor		o —> X		

o = current position
x = degree of commitment required

You can see that the chief executive is currently not committed, and, being a key figure, it would desirable for this person to lead the change and make it happen. The health visitor only needs to move a short way to be in the most desirable position, while the GP needs to step back a little, from leading the change to just supporting it.

Three-phase model (Lewin, 1951)

This works by:

1 **Unfreezing** – get people to accept that there is a need for change. Take care to recognise people's past achievements though, allowing them to have pride in (and even 'grieve' for) the old ways before proceeding to the next stage.
2 **Moving** – put the new changes into effect. This may need careful planning and monitoring. Resistance may start to appear, so be prepared to make the changes gradually if necessary.
3 **Refreezing** – new changes become normal practice. Old ways are firmly discouraged.

Six methods for overcoming resistance (Kotter and Schlesinger, 1979)

Various methods are suggested for dealing with resistance to change:

1 Education and communication – educate people beforehand.
2 Participation and involvement – involve others at the outset.
3 Facilitation and support – provide training in new working methods.
4 Negotiation and agreement – agree incentives to adopt new methods.
5 Manipulation and co-optation – use methods to influence others.
6 Explicit and implicit coercion – make threats to gain compliance.

Obviously the last two methods are unlikely to be appropriate! Always consider your strategy carefully, avoiding a disjointed approach, and be as open as possible about your plans.

Audit terminology

Audit

A way of formally evaluating care by setting standards, measuring activity and implementing change.

Audit cycle

The process of carrying out audits and repeating them to continually assess the effectiveness of the care being audited.

Clinical audit

Audit involving personnel from more than one profession (e.g. GPs and practice nurses).

Clinical governance

A framework through which NHS organisations are accountable for continuously improving the quality of their services, and safeguarding high standards of care by creating an environment in which excellence in clinical care will flourish (Department of Health, 1998).

Commission for Health Improvement (CHI)

An independent organisation, which reports to the Department of Health. It was established to improve the quality of patient care in the NHS. CHI aims to raise standards by assessing every NHS organisation and making its findings public, investigating when there is serious failure, checking that the NHS is following national guidelines and advising the NHS on best practice.

Criterion

Something that can be counted or measured in order to assess the quality of care.

Effectiveness

How much benefit is being achieved.

Efficiency

The extent to which benefits are achieved without incurring unnecessary expenditure.

Evaluation

Process of determining the effectiveness, efficiency and acceptability of planned actions in achieving stated objectives.

Evidence-based medicine

Clinical practice which is based on valid, up-to-date research that delivers proven benefits to patients.

Explicit

Clearly and unambiguously stated.

GP

General practitioner – clinician delivering primary healthcare.

Hawthorne effect

A theory that people work better when they know their activities are being monitored.

Implicit

Implied, rather than being clearly stated.

Interface audit

Audits which evaluate activities carried out by more than one agency (e.g. primary and secondary care).

Likert scale

A method of answering a question by selecting one of a range of numbers (e.g. 1 = excellent; 2 = good; 3 = fair; 4 = bad; 5 = very bad).

Medical audit

Audit which is carried out by doctors only. This has now been largely replaced by clinical audit, involving personnel from other professions and disciplines.

MAAG

Acronym for Medical Audit Advisory Group. These groups were established in the early 1990s to encourage all GP practices to carry out audit. Some still exist, though most have disappeared, and many primary care trusts (PCTs) have their own audit staff.

Methodology

Instructions describing how an audit will be carried out.

Multiprofessional audit

Audit involving personnel from more than one profession or discipline. It is the same as clinical audit.

National Service Frameworks (NSFs)

A collection of evidence-based documents defining national standards of service which should be provided for patients with certain conditions or in certain groups (e.g. diabetes, coronary heart disease, older people).

Outcome

The results of healthcare, especially those which have an impact on the health of patients.

Primary care

The part of healthcare which is delivered through GP practices, rather than hospitals.

Primary care trusts (PCTs)

These are local groups of healthcare professionals, working in partnership with other organisations and agencies. The function of PCTs is to improve the health of the community, develop primary and community health services, and commission secondary care services. PCTs are responsible for delivering better healthcare to their local population, and carry out many of the functions previously performed by old health authorities. They can also provide a range of community health services.

Process

The activities of those involved in the care of patients.

Prospective audit

Audit based on present and future events, rather than what has happened in the past.

Protocol

A detailed written plan for carrying out an audit, containing the audit's aims, criteria, standards and methodology.

Reliability

The consistency or dependability with which an instrument measures what it is supposed to measure. *See also* Validity.

Retrospective audit

Audit based on past events.

Secondary care

The part of healthcare which is delivered through hospitals.

Significant event audit

Audit involving the retrospective examination of circumstances which may have resulted in an unsatisfactory outcome (e.g. suicide, missed diagnosis of cancer).

Standard

An expression of how often a criterion should be achieved.

Structure

The resources that facilitate the process of care (e.g. buildings, equipment or salaries of personnel).

Tertiary care

The part of healthcare which is delivered through agencies other than GP practices and hospitals, such as community care and mental healthcare.

Validity

The accuracy with which an instrument measures what it is supposed to measure. *See also* Reliability.

3

Searching for evidence

We have already discussed the need for standards to be based on clinically effective practice. This is practice which is based on valid, up-to-date research that delivers proven benefits to patients, and is also known as evidence-based medicine. A dazzling array of information sources are available, which can be used to find research papers, reviews of evidence, health economic analyses and other documents.

But how do you go about finding such evidence? This can seem very daunting, as there are so many possible sources of information. This chapter aims to help you think about what you need to do when searching for evidence, and provides some tips on how to search effectively, along with details of a few useful websites to get you started.

It is vital to know exactly what you want to search for, so you can find exactly what you require. For example, if you are looking for evidence on 'diabetes', are you interested in patients with type I, type II or any type of diabetes? If your audit will exclusively study Asian children with type I diabetes, your search *may* need to be focused on this specific patient group, to avoid finding superfluous information (as data on middle-aged Caucasians with type II diabetes may be inappropriate in this case). Also, diabetes is sometimes known as 'diabetes mellitus', so it is worth finding out whether the subject of your search is known by any other names, or is spelled differently in other English-speaking countries (for example in the USA, 'oesophagus' is spelled 'esophagus', and 'anaemia' is spelled 'anemia'). Also drugs are sometimes known by different proprietary names (e.g. Riluzole's proprietary name is Rilutek®, and the proprietary name of the levonorgestrel-releasing intrauterine system is Mirena®). If you are aiming to find a wide range of evidence on your subject, you may need to search on every possible permutation.

To make things even more complicated, much valuable information never gets published. This may be because investigators abandon projects before they are completed, or never get around to writing them up and submitting for publication, and journals may reject submitted papers for many reasons. Unpublished evidence can be useful, and should not therefore be ignored.

Some of the information you find may be in languages other than English. Although this presents obvious difficulties, don't assume that such information will not be useful, just because you cannot read it. Abstracts of foreign papers sometimes appear in English, and you may know individuals who can translate the papers for you. Also, Internet sites such as the AltaVista search engine have a really useful translation facility (online at http://babel.altavista.com/tr?) which can be used for blocks of text.

It is necessary to find a balance between spending a substantial amount of time trying to find *every* piece of evidence on a subject (important if you are carrying out a large review of evidence to make a decision about a treatment's effectiveness, for example), and doing a less systematic search in a more manageable time frame.

So where can you look for evidence, and how should you search for it? You might like to consider the following:

- Decide where you are going to search – electronic databases, appropriate journals, conference proceedings, other sources.
- If using an electronic search engine, formulate a strategy for finding what you need – key words; alternative names, terms and spellings.
- Seek advice and assistance from librarians.
- Identify and contact subject experts/authors of studies in the subject area. They are often happy to help, and a goldmine of valuable information – especially unpublished data.

Here are some tips on using electronic databases:

- Start with subject of interest, then convert each element into a series of keywords. Think of synonyms/alternative spellings (e.g. neurone/neuron)
- Find nearest equivalent indexing terms (MeSH headings – for MEDLINE and Cochrane Library) – look at those in any papers you have already found
- Some databases allow MeSH (Medical Subject Headings, e.g. anaemia – hypochronic)

- Use AND/OR (e.g. 'Asian AND diabetes' gives you everyone who is Asian AND has diabetes)
- Textwords (words appearing in title or abstract, e.g. iron deficiency anaemia)
- Use a combination of textword and indexing terms
- Consider using published pre-defined search strategies ('filters')
- Compromise between 'sensitivity' (getting everything relevant) and 'specificity' (proportion of hits to hits and misses); to be comprehensive, you must sacrifice specificity
- If too many records are retrieved, narrow the search:
  - use more specific or more relevant textwords
  - use MeSH terms rather than textwords
  - select specific subheadings with MeSH terms
- If too few records are retrieved, widen the search:
  - use more terms
  - use 'explosion' feature (if available)
  - select all subheadings with MeSH terms

You might find the following selection of electronic databases and search engines useful:

MEDLINE – covers the whole field of medical information. Available from several sources (e.g. via Ovid or Silverplatter in medical libraries or by corporate subscription) or at http://www.nlm.nih.gov/ or via the BMJ website: http://bmj.com/misc/medline.shtml

Search strategies for identifying reviews in MEDLINE at: http://www.york.ac.uk/inst/crd/search.htm

NHS Centre for Reviews and Dissemination: http://nhscrd.york.ac.uk/

Cochrane Library of Systematic Reviews: http://www.nelh.nhs.uk/cochrane.asp

UK Health Technology Assessment Programme: http://www.hta.nhsweb.nhs.uk/main.htm

National Research Register: http://www.doh.gov.uk/research/nrr.htm

National electronic Library for Health: http://www.nelh.nhs.uk/

Regional Department of Research and Development: http://www.doh.gov.uk/research/wmro/

Bandolier – newsletter of literature on healthcare effectiveness: http://www.jr2.ox.ac.uk/bandolier/

BMJ website – electronic version of all BMJ issues since 1994, plus a useful search/archiving facility: http://www.bmj.com/

Department of Health: www.doh.gov.uk

Official documents: www.official-documents.co.uk/

Office for National Statistics (ONS): http://www.statistics.gov.uk/

Other databases:
EMBASE: http://www.embase.com/ for registered users
Science Citation Index – accessible by licensed institutions
CINAHL – accessible by licensed institutions

Internet search engines (e.g. Google http://www.google.co.uk/; AltaVista http://uk.altavista.com/)

4

Introduction to Epi Info

What is Epi Info?

Epi Info is a series of computer programs (Dean *et al.*, 1995), incorporating a database program. Computer databases store information rather like cards in a card-index system. Each individual card can hold several pieces of information. When you want to retrieve the information, you can either find the appropriate card, or look through several cards and make a note of the details required. For instance, a simple index card might look like this:

```
Patient ID _____

Date of birth ____/____/_____

Gender _____

BMI _____
```

The card contains four items of information – *patient ID, date of birth, gender* and *BMI.*

- The lines on the card represent the places where the information is actually recorded, and can be referred to as information FIELDS.
- The words *'patient ID'*, *'date of birth'*, *'gender'* and *'BMI'* can be referred to as FIELD NAMES. They act as labels – without them, you do not know what kind of information is recorded on any particular line.
- Each card can be referred to as a RECORD, and a collection of records can be called a FILE.
- A computer database consists of *files*, all containing a number of *records*, each of which stores *fields* of information.

Five steps to using Epi Info

1 Create your questionnaire or form using EPED.
2 Convert the form to a record file, using ENTER.
3 If required, use CHECK to set up legal values, jump fields, etc (these will be explained later).
4 Input the data in ENTER.
5 Analyse the data in ANALYSIS by producing graphs, tables, lists, etc.

Example

If you are creating a computer database based on the above card:

1 First, you need to create a master document containing all the required fields, each preceded by a field name. In Epi Info, you would use EPED to create this master document.
2 You may wish to ensure that 'age' is entered on every computer record, and not missed during data entry. This would be set up in CHECK.
3 If 100 people each write their own details on one of the above cards, you will have 100 records to enter onto your database, each containing four fields. You would use ENTER to input the information.
4 When you have inputted all of the data, you can ask the computer to look at particular fields of information and, for instance, produce:
   - a list of IDs
   - a table showing BMI values
   - a pie chart showing genders.
   You would use Epi Info's ANALYSIS program to produce these.

How Epi Info can help with clinical audit

Epi Info can be an invaluable aid to carrying out clinical audit. This is mainly because it does much of the hard work of audit for you – namely making it easy to enter and store your data, then analysing it and calculating the statistics. These activities are probably the most feared and hated aspects of audit. Most of us are reasonably happy to think up subjects for audit, set standards and even collect some data. But the thought of having to sort through reams of paper to find out what is going on, then work out statistics to describe them accurately does not always fall within our comfort zone.

Using Epi Info can help to free you of this drudgery for ever. While having an appreciation of basic statistics (*see* Chapter 7) will help you to decide which methods to use, the software will do the rest. Take the time to learn how to use Epi Info, and it will repay you over and over again, saving time on every project.

- It is extremely quick and simple to enter data.
- There are special facilities which help to make your data entry more accurate.
- Once data are entered, they can be analysed instantly.
- Data analysis is fast and simple.
- Sums, percentages and other statistics are calculated automatically.
- Many statistical tests can be carried out (such as *t*-tests, chi-squared and more).
- You can easily limit your analysis to specific groups (e.g. females who are over 30 and smoke).
- These groups can easily be compared with each other – something which cannot easily be achieved with spreadsheets (e.g. against males who are aged over 30 and smoke).

Using Epi Info will help you to plan better audit projects. The process of creating data collection forms, setting up fields and analysing the data will make you think more carefully about what data to collect, how to collect them and how they will be analysed in future audits. It is easier, cheaper and more practical to use than many other computer packages. Whatever kind of audit or survey you are going to carry out, Epi Info will save you a great deal of time and grief.

Summary of programs included in Epi Info v6.04

- **EPED** – a basic word processor for creating questionnaires and data collection forms.
- **ENTER** – automatically produces a data file from questionnaires/ forms created in EPED or another word processor. Saves information

to a disk. Allows revision of file format even after records have been entered.

- **ENTER/X** – identical in use to ENTER, but uses higher memory, allowing larger questionnaires and complex data validation codes to be used. You only need to use this option if you are unable to use ENTER because of memory limitations (i.e. if ENTER requires more memory than the usual DOS limit of 640K).
- **ANALYSIS** – produces tables, lists, graphs, cross-tabulations and other types of result. Records can be selected or sorted in various ways. Data items spread over several files can be linked and analysed as a single unit.
- **CHECK** – sets ranges, legal values, skip patterns and automatic coding. These can help when inputting data in the ENTER program.
- **IMPORT** – imports files from other systems for use within Epi Info.
- **EXPORT** – converts data files from Epi Info format into 12 other formats (including Lotus 1-2-3 and dBASE) for a variety of database and statistics programs.
- **MERGE** – allows you to combine data files and update old records with new data.
- **STATCALC** – calculates statistics, such as sample size, single and stratified chi-square for trend, and single and stratified 2×2 tables.
- **CSAMPLE** – allows you to analyse data from complex sample surveys.
- **EPITABLE** – calculates various epidemiological statistics.
- **EPINUT** – processes files to add nutritional calculations.
- **VALIDATE** – compares any two files in Epi Info format, and reports any differences.
- **EXAMPLE PROGRAMS** – a collection of sample programs is available.
- **HELP and TUTORIALS** – on-screen help and a complete interactive tutorial are provided, to introduce the features of EPED, ENTER and ANALYSIS.
- **MANUAL** – the full manual is available on-line, with index features.

Facts about Epi Info

- It is a series of computer programs produced by The Division of Surveillance & Epidemiology, Epidemiology Program Office, Centers for Disease Control and Prevention (CDC), Atlanta, Georgia, in collaboration with the Global Programme on AIDS, WHO, Geneva, Switzerland.

- The programs are *not* subject to copyright. Making copies for others is permitted and encouraged.
- Epi Info runs on almost any IBM compatible computer (PC). The minimum requirement is the PC-DOS or MS-DOS operating system, 640K of RAM and at least one floppy disk drive.
- Graphs and text can be printed with a range of printers, including IBM or Epson-compatible printers, or with Hewlett-Packard-compatible laser printers, plotters and postscript printers.
- Data files can consist of as many records as DOS and your disk storage can handle (billions). A questionnaire can have up to 500 lines or approximately 20 screens. The number of variables is not limited, except that they must fit in the 500 lines. The maximum length for a text variable is 80 characters. The maximum number of fields is 120. The total length of variables in one file must not exceed 2048 characters.
- Epi Info version 6.04d only requires around 9 Mbyte of disk space.
- The software can be downloaded from the Epi Info website – see instructions on p. 44.

Installing Epi Info v6.04d on your computer

Epi Info can be installed from CD-ROM (supplied), floppy disk or direct from the Internet. Installation is different for each type of media, so separate instructions are shown for each. A small number of minor problems can arise when using Epi Info under certain versions of Windows, and details are given of how these might be overcome.

A number of example Epi Info files are supplied, which are used in certain sections of this book. These do not automatically install with Epi Info, and have to be copied over manually. Again, full instructions of how to do this are given.

Installing Epi Info from CD-ROM (supplied with this book)

1 Open Windows Explorer.
2 Click on D (or the letter that represents your CD-ROM drive. Depending on which version of Windows you are using, this might be located within 'My Computer').
3 Double-click on the '**Install.exe**' file to load the program.
4 Follow instructions on-screen. Your SOURCE drive will probably be **D**; DESTINATION drive will probably be **C**.

Press ⟨ENTER⟩ if the source drive letter shown is correct. If it is not correct, type a different letter, followed by ⟨ENTER⟩.

Answer the following questions:

- Does your computer have a *removable* drive? Type N if it does not (your computer will almost certainly *not* have a removable drive).
- Press ⟨ENTER⟩ if you want a 'normal' installation. 'Normal' means that Epi Info will be installed into a directory called C:\EPI6 (recommended). If you really do not want this, press ⟨Esc⟩.
- Would you like to INSTALL the system for use, or COPY it for further distribution? (Type I to install Epi Info.)
- What kind of video board is in your computer? (Accept the option given, then press **F4**, unless you are sure that your video board is different.)
- Select the driver(s) for your printer(s) by highlighting the printer type then pressing the space bar on your keyboard. Continue this process for any additional printer drivers, then press **F4** to continue.
- It is suggested that you allow all of the program groups to be installed – press **F4** to accept this.
- Press ⟨ENTER⟩ to complete the installation process. You will then see various files scrolling down your screen.
- It is advisable for you to allow Epi Info to edit your AUTOEXEC.BAT and CONFIG.SYS files – just type Y when prompted.

5 Press ⟨ENTER⟩ to leave the installation program when prompted.
6 To create a shortcut, use Windows Explorer to find the newly created EPI6 folder on your hard drive (usually at C:\EPI6).
7 In the EPI6 folder, find the **EPI6.EXE** icon. Right-click on this icon, and select 'create shortcut'.
8 A new icon called 'shortcut to EPI6' will be created. Drag this new icon to your desktop.
9 Double click the icon to start Epi Info.

WARNING

The INSTALL program will create a subdirectory called EPI6 on your hard disk.

It is advisable for you to check that you do not already have a subdirectory with the name EPI6 on your hard disk.

To find out, look in the C: directory in Windows Explorer, or type **DIR/W** at the C:> prompt, and see if **[EPI6]** appears in the listing on the screen.

If it *is* listed then you should rename it (or create a new subdirectory with a different name and copy your files to it). Otherwise Epi Info will not install, or will overwrite your existing EPI6 subdirectory.

Epi Info version 6.04d is Year 2000 compliant.

Installing Epi Info from floppy disks (not supplied with this book)

DOS	Windows 3.1/3.11	Windows 95/98/2000/XP, etc.
1 Exit any programs currently running on your computer, so that you get a blank screen which just displays **C:>**	1 Insert Epi Info v6.04d disk no.1 into the floppy drive on your computer	1 Insert Epi Info v6.04d disk no.1 into the floppy drive on your computer
2 Insert Epi Info v6.04d disk no.1 into the floppy drive on your computer	2 Select FILE (In top left-hand area of the screen), and click your left mouse button	2 Click on the **START** icon
3 Type `A:install` then press ⟨ENTER⟩	3 From the FILE menu select RUN and click	3 Click on 'RUN'
4 Follow instruction 5 (below) onwards	4 In the 'Command Line' box, type `A:install` then click on 'OK' and follow instruction 5 (below) onwards	4 In the box on the screen, type `A:install` then click on 'OK' and follow instruction 5 (below) onwards

5 Your SOURCE drive will probably be **A**, DESTINATION drive will probably be **C**. Press ⟨ENTER⟩ if the source drive letter shown is correct. If it is not correct, type a different letter, followed by ⟨ENTER⟩. Answer the following questions:

- Does your computer have a *removable* drive? Type N if it does not (your computer will almost certainly *not* have a removable drive).
- Press ⟨ENTER⟩ if you want a 'normal' installation. 'Normal' means that Epi Info will be installed into a directory called C:\EPI6 (recommended). If you really do not want this, press ⟨Esc⟩.

- Would you like to INSTALL the system for use, or COPY it for further distribution? (Type I to install Epi Info.)
- What kind of video board is in your computer? (Accept the option given, then press **F4**, unless you are sure that your video board is different.)
- Select the driver(s) for your printer(s) by highlighting the printer type then pressing the space bar on your keyboard. Continue this process for any additional printer drivers, then press **F4** to continue.
- It is suggested that you allow all of the program groups to be installed – press **F4** to accept this.
- Press ⟨ENTER⟩ to complete the installation process. You will then see various files scrolling down your screen.
- It is advisable for you to allow Epi Info to edit your AUTOEXEC.BAT and CONFIG.SYS files – just type Y when prompted.

6 When the following appears on screen, insert disk no. 2 and press ⟨ENTER⟩.

```
Group 7: NUTRITIONAL ANTHROPOMETRY
   Please insert the disk containing group 7 into drive A:
     and press ⟨ENTER⟩ (or press ⟨ESC⟩ to skip group 7)
         (Group 7 is probably on the next disk)
```

7 When the following appears on screen, insert disk no. 3 and press ⟨ENTER⟩.

```
Group 12: NETSS: Model Surveillance System
   Please insert the disk containing group 12 into
     drive A:
         and press ⟨ENTER⟩ (or press ⟨ESC⟩ to skip group 12)
            (Group 12 is probably on the next disk)
```

8 Press ⟨ENTER⟩ to leave the installation program when prompted. (DOS only: at the A:\> prompt, type **C:** and press ⟨ENTER⟩.)

Downloading Epi Info from the Internet

- Go to website address: http://www.cdc.gov/epiinfo/EI6dnjp.htm.
- Click on the 'Epi Info 6 for DOS' icon and click on 'downloads'.

- To get a complete installation package, download and run all three self-expanding, compressed files to a temporary directory:
  - EPI604_1.EXE (file size = 1 367 649 bytes)
  - EPI604_2.EXE (file size = 1 341 995 bytes)
  - EPI604_3.EXE (file size = 1 360 925 bytes).
- Then run INSTALL.EXE to install the software. You can do this by viewing the downloaded files using Windows Explorer or Winfile, then double clicking on the file called 'INSTALL.EXE'.
- Follow the installation instructions from 5 onwards, as shown in the previous section.

Accessing the Epi Info menu

Note – you will not need this section if you have installed Epi Info from the CD-ROM, and followed the instructions on p. 41.

Accessing Epi Info from DOS

Exit any programs currently running on your computer, so that you get a blank screen which just displays **C:>**.

1 Type **CD\EPI6** then press ⟨ENTER⟩ (ensure you press EPI6, *not* EP16).
2 Type **EPI6** then press ⟨ENTER⟩.

Accessing Epi Info from Windows 3.1/3.11/95/98/2000/XP

Double-click on the Epi Info icon. Use the instructions below to set up the icon for the first time. Epi Info v6.04d usually runs perfectly well under the above versions of Windows.

Setting up an Epi Info icon

Setting up an Epi Info Icon in Windows 3.1/3.11

1 Get into the Windows program manager, and open the program group you wish to run Epi Info from (e.g. 'Main').
2 Select FILE (in top left-hand area of the screen), and click your left mouse button.
3 From the FILE menu, select RUN, and click.
4 In the 'Command Line' box, type **C:\EPI6\SETUP.EXE**.
5 Click on 'OK'.
6 Click on 'OK' again, and a program group called 'Epi Info v6' will be created.

7 Highlight the 'EPI6 MENU' icon, and double click on it or press ⟨ENTER⟩ to access Epi Info.

Setting up an Epi Info icon in Windows 95/98/2000/XP

1 In Windows Explorer, click on the newly created EPI6 folder.
2 Find the EPI6.exe icon and right-click on it.
3 Select 'Create Shortcut' – an icon called 'Shortcut to EPI6' will be created in the EPI6 folder.
4 Drag 'Shortcut to EPI6' from Explorer to your desktop.
5 Double-click the shortcut to start EPI6.

Screen display problems

When running Epi Info within certain versions of Windows, it may initially be displayed in a small window on the screen. If this happens, clicking on the ⊞ icon may solve the problem, by making it fill the screen.
  If the ⊞ icon does not appear on your screen, try the following:

1 Exit from the small Epi Info window (press **F10**).
2 Find the Epi Info icon on your desktop.
3 Click on it, using the right-hand mouse button.
4 Click on PROPERTIES – this brings up the EPI6.EXE properties window.
5 In this window, click on PROGRAM.
6 Look for RUN, and click on the scroll bar alongside it.
7 Select MAXIMISED.
8 Now click on the SCREEN section of the window.
9 Under USAGE, click the circle next to FULL-SCREEN.
10 Click APPLY (to the bottom right of the window).
11 Click OK.
12 Now double-click on the Epi Info icon.
13 The Epi Info screen should now occupy the whole of your screen.

The above instructions tend to produce better results with standard PC monitors than with laptop computers. Even if this does not work for your computer, the small display should be perfectly readable.

Copying the example Epi Info files

As previously mentioned, a number of example Epi Info files are supplied on the CD-ROM, and these are used in certain sections of this book. They do not automatically install with Epi Info, and have to be copied over manually. To do this, follow these instructions:

1 Open Windows Explorer.
2 Find the EPI6 directory, that was created when Epi Info was installed (this may be located within 'My Computer').
3 Click on the D drive (or the drive that represents your CD-ROM drive).
4 Click on the directory called 'Example Files'.
5 Copy each file in the 'Example Files' directory over to your 'EPI6' directory. (*Hint*: to select all of the files, press and hold down the **Ctrl** key, then click on each of the files once. Alternatively, click 'Edit', then 'Select All'.) Then click on the highlighted block of files using the left-hand mouse button, and drag them over to the EPI6 directory (make sure that the EPI6 directory is displayed on your screen before you drag the files over). Alternatively, when you have highlighted all of the files, click the right-hand mouse button – this will bring up a menu. Click on 'Copy' on the menu. Next, locate and click on the EPI6 directory, and click on the right-hand mouse button – this will bring up another menu. Finally, click on 'Paste' on the menu. This will copy the files over.

The Epi Info menu

The Epi Info menu looks like this:

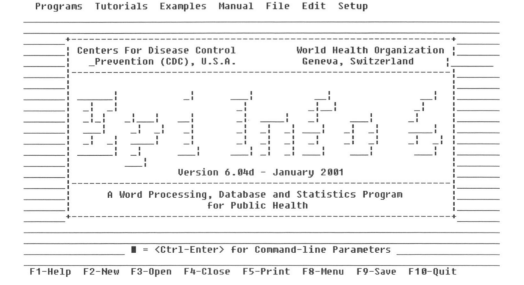

```
 Programs  Tutorials  Examples  Manual  File  Edit  Setup
```

Main menu items are located along the top of the screen. To move around the screen, use the mouse or arrow keys. The mouse can also be used with some of Epi Info's programs, but with others the arrow keys ($\leftarrow$, $\uparrow$, $\downarrow$, $\rightarrow$) and function keys (**F1** to **F12**) are used instead. The ⟨**ENTER**⟩ key is also frequently used – this is the key marked $\hookleftarrow$.

Various menus are used within Epi Info's programs. If you open one in error, it can be closed by pressing the **Esc** key.

Click on a highlighted item, or press ⟨ENTER⟩ to view its contents. As each item is highlighted, a submenu drops down, allowing you to select further options. As you move around, either up or down, a message on the bottom line of the screen displays a brief description of the option highlighted. To open a particular option, simply press ⟨ENTER⟩ or click the mouse button.

The most commonly used programs are contained in the PROGRAMS menu, at the top left-hand corner of the screen. Programs such as EPED, ENTER, ANALYSIS and CHECK can be found here.

To close Epi Info, press **F10** (or select QUIT from the FILE menu).

EPED

When EPED is accessed through the PROGRAMS menu, this screen will appear:

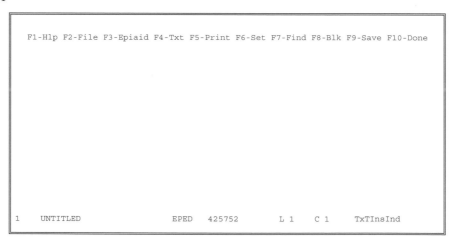

```
F1-Hlp F2-File F3-Epiaid F4-Txt F5-Print F6-Set F7-Find F8-Blk F9-Save F10-Done




















1    UNTITLED              EPED   425752      L 1    C 1     TxTInsInd
```

EPED is used for creating questionnaires and data collection forms. It can also serve as a *very* basic word processor.

Documents produced within EPED serve as 'master sheets' for inputting information at a later stage.

Opening files in EPED

If you wish to open an existing file, press **F2** and select 'OPEN FILE THIS WINDOW', then press ⟨ENTER⟩. Type the whole filename into the box on screen and press ⟨ENTER⟩, or if you cannot remember it, press ⟨ENTER⟩ for a menu of all available files (EPED files end in **.QES**).

If, however, you wish to start a new file, simply begin typing onto the screen.

Fields and field names

So that Epi Info can store and analyse the data you will eventually be inputting, it is necessary to create a FIELD for every item of information that you wish to collect and analyse. Epi Info only analyses areas of the document which you have designated as fields, so you are free to type other information anywhere else on the page (e.g. a title, instructions or an explanation).

As outlined on p. 38, each field should be prefixed with a FIELD NAME. This can be up to ten characters in length. If it is any longer, Epi Info will just use the first ten characters. For instance, a field name could be 'AGE', 'SEX' or 'HOW MANY?'.

If you want to enter a particularly long piece of text in front of a field, such as 'How many cigarettes do you smoke each day?', you can put significant words inside curly brackets (e.g. How many {cigarettes} do you smoke each day?). In this example, Epi Info recognises 'cigarettes' as the field name. *Note*: certain words (e.g. 'When', 'What' or 'Did') are ignored by the ANALYSIS program if you try to include them as field names.

After entering the field name, the actual *field* can be created. There are several types available – to use them, press and hold down the **Ctrl** button and type: **QQ** (alternatively, you could press **F4** [Txt] and then ⟨ENTER⟩ [Questions]). This menu then appears on your screen:

```
      Epi Info Questions

   ------------------
   ##
   <A      >
   <Y>
   <mm/dd/yyyy>
   <mm/dd/yy>
   <mm/dd>
   <dd/mm/yyyy>
   <dd/mm/yy>
   <dd/mm>
   <phonenum>
   <long distance>
   <today>
   <today/yy>
   <today/yyyy>
   <idnum>
```

_ _ _ _ _ _ _ _ _ _ _ _ _ _ *Free text*

This type of field accepts letters, words, numbers or other characters. It is particularly useful for recording responses to open questions (e.g. 'What do you think of our {car-parking} facilities?'). When you select this field type, a box appears on the screen, prompting you to specify how many characters the text field should consist of, up to a maximum of 80.

Numeric field

Use this field if you wish to record numbers. Letters or other characters are not accepted if any attempt is made to input them in the ENTER program. Upon selecting this field, a box appears on the screen, prompting you to specify how many digits you would like the field to consist of, both before and after the decimal point. If you do not require digits after the decimal point, press ⟨ENTER⟩ to ignore.

For instance, if you want to record people's ages, you will probably need only three digits, with no decimal point – '###'. If, however, you are recording weight in kilograms, you may need three digits before the decimal point, and two after it – '###.##'.

⟨A⟩ *Upper-case field*

This is identical to the Free text field, except that letters and characters are automatically converted to upper case. This is useful, since Epi Info is case-sensititve (e.g. it will treat the words 'nurse', 'Nurse' and 'NURSE' as separate entries, which would be misleading in an analysis). Having all entries in upper case helps you to avoid this problem by standardising the case of your entries.

⟨Y⟩ *Yes/No field*

You can only enter 'Y' or 'N' is this field, as a response to a 'yes or no' question.

⟨mm/dd/yyyy⟩, ⟨mm/dd/yy⟩, ⟨mm/dd⟩, ⟨dd/mm/yyyy⟩, ⟨dd/mm/yy⟩, ⟨dd/mm⟩ *Date fields*

Allows you to enter dates in a choice of formats. English formats are usually either ⟨dd/mm/yyyy⟩, ⟨dd/mm/yy⟩ or ⟨dd/mm⟩. When dates are being inputted, only the actual numbers need to be entered – the 'slash marks' ('/') in between are added automatically. The program does *not* allow you to enter invalid dates (e.g. 94/56/12).

⟨phone num⟩ *Eight-digit telephone number*

Accepts eight-digit numbers only.

⟨long distance⟩ *Long-distance telephone number*

Accepts 13-digit numbers only.

⟨today⟩, ⟨today/yy⟩, ⟨today/yyyy⟩ *Today's date*

Inserts the date (which your computer acknowledges as being today's) in one of three formats. This field can either be used to denote the date on which the data were entered, or the date on which the record was last updated. You do not have to input any information for this field; pressing ⟨ENTER⟩ automatically inserts the date.

⟨idnum⟩ *Automatically incremented field*

Provides each record with a unique identification number. This number is automatically inserted by the program when inputting data, starting at number 1 on the first record and incrementing by one for each subsequent record.

Note: the number of fields you include in a document is limited to 120, and they must fit into a maximum of 500 lines, and the total number of characters within all the fields must not exceed 2048 (e.g. you can have no more than 25 free text fields, if each one each contains 80 characters). If more fields are required than can be accommodated, it is advisable to create extra *files* to store the data.

Typing and editing text

You can type words, numbers and characters onto the screen in the same way as you would with a word processor.

Here is a list of some commands used in EPED:

- To add a field, press and hold **Ctrl** and type QQ.
- Delete characters using the **Back Space (←)** or **Del** key.
- Press **Ctrl** and **Y** simultaneously to delete a whole line.

- Press **F4** for a menu of text options (Format Paragraph, Type Style, Undelete, etc.).
- Press **F6** for a menu of setup options (Page Breaks, Justification, Margins, Tabs, etc.)
- Press **F8** for a menu of blocking options (Begin Block, End Block, Copy Block to Here, Move Block to Here, Delete Block, etc.).
- Press **Esc** to remove any menus you have called up, if they are not required.
- Boxes and areas of shading can be added to your document. Press the **Scroll Lock** key to see instructions for this facility.

Printing the document

If you would like a printout of the file:

1 Ensure that you have a suitable printer connected to your computer.
2 Press **F5**.
3 A box appears, allowing you to view and amend the printer setup if necessary. To amend the setup, highlight the item to change, then press ⟨ENTER⟩.
4 When the setup is satisfactory, highlight '**print file now**'.
5 Press ⟨ENTER⟩.

Saving the file

It is wise to save your document at regular intervals while you are working on it, so that you do not lose all the information if there is a power failure or some other problem occurs.

- If you are saving the file for the *first time*, press **F9** and a box appears on the screen, prompting you to insert a name. Type in a filename, followed by .QES (remember the full stop!).

Note: all documents created within EPED for subsequent data entry and analysis *must* be suffixed with .QES.

- Just press **F9** to save an *existing* file.

Converting the file into ENTRY format

When all the required field names and fields have been entered, you need to convert the file into a format suitable for data entry. Follow these steps:

1 Save the file, by pressing **F9**.
2 Press **F10** to exit EPED.
3 Access the ENTRY menu (from the PROGRAM menu on the main screen).
4 Type a filename (it is a good idea to use the same filename as your .QES file), then press ⟨ENTER⟩.
5 Type **2**, and press ⟨ENTER⟩.
6 Type in the filename of your .QES file and press ⟨ENTER⟩ (press **F9** for a list of files if you cannot remember the filename).
7 Press ⟨ENTER⟩ again to confirm.

The file is displayed in data entry format, and you can begin entering data straight away. The ENTRY file created has the same filename, but ends in .REC (signifying that it is a **record file**).

Changing the file at a later stage

One feature of Epi Info is that you can go back into EPED and change a .QES file, even after you have started to input data in the ENTER program.
  If you wish to do this, follow these steps:

1 Go into EPED, and open the file you want to change.
2 Make your changes.
3 Press **F9** to save the file.
4 Press **F10** to exit EPED.
5 Go into the ENTER menu.
6 Enter the name of the .REC file, and press ⟨ENTER⟩.
7 Type 3, and press ⟨ENTER⟩.
8 Type the filename of your revised .QES file, and press ⟨ENTER⟩.
9 Press ⟨ENTER⟩ again to confirm.

Various text then scrolls down the screen, and you are informed that all records have been successfully merged. *Note*: *never* try to edit a .REC file using EPED. If you use this facility to change a field that already contains data, the data that has already been entered into the field may be lost.

Exiting EPED

Press **F10** to exit the program.

CHECK

This program can simplify data entry in various ways. A check file can be set up on any file with a .REC suffix. This check file is saved with the same filename, but ending in .CHK (a check file created for PATIENTS.REC would be saved as PATIENTS.CHK).

Setting up CHECK functions on a file

1 Make sure the file has been saved in the ENTER program (i.e. ends in .REC).
2 Access the main EPI menu.
3 Select CHECK from the PROGRAMS menu.
4 Press ⟨ENTER⟩.
5 Type the name of the .REC file.
6 Press ⟨ENTER⟩.

Your form then appears on the screen.

Some available CHECK facilities

- **Legal values** – only certain entries are accepted (e.g. if you set up a field for the names of local consultants, it will only allow those individuals' names to be entered in that field).
    Follow these steps:
    1 Place the cursor in the field required.
    2 Type the word, letter, character or number that you wish to be accepted.
    3 Press **F6** ('legal').
    4 Repeat steps 2 and 3 for all other words, letters, characters or numbers required.
    When entering the data, all legal entries are displayed near the bottom of the screen. Pressing **F9** displays a list of legal entries, which can be selected and entered by highlighting the entry required, then pressing ⟨ENTER⟩. This function is useful, since it saves you having to type the entry in full, and also helps avoid spelling mistakes.
- **Must enter** – does not allow an entry to be skipped, ensuring that data are always entered in a particular field. Use the following steps to set this up:
    1 Place the cursor in the field required.
    2 Press **F4**.
    Pressing **F4** again on the same field removes the 'must enter' condition.
- **Skip patterns** – in some circumstances, one or more fields can be skipped, depending on the answer to a prior question. For example, if one field asks whether a particular respondent smokes, and the next five ask about his/her smoking habits, a response of 'no' to the first question means that the following five fields will be left blank. It would

therefore simplify data entry if a response of 'no' automatically moved the cursor to a question further down the form, removing the need to press ⟨ENTER⟩ to skip over the unnecessary fields.

To set up skip patterns:

1 Place the cursor in the appropriate field (e.g. 'Do you smoke?').
2 Type **N** if you want to skip the next field on a response of 'N'.
3 Press **F7** ('jump').
4 Place the cursor in the destination field (where you want to skip *to*).
5 Press **F7** again.

In this example, an answer of 'N' to 'Do you smoke?' automatically causes the cursor to skip to the destination field. If the answer is 'Y', the cursor moves to the next field as usual.

Exiting CHECK

After you have set up all the required CHECK functions:

1 Press **F10** to quit.
2 Type Y to save the information.
3 You will be returned to the EPI main menu.

ENTER

When ENTER is accessed through the PROGRAMS menu, this screen will appear:

```
Version 6.04d - (real mode)          Enter                    January 2001

                       Data file  ( .REC) :


            ┌──────────────────────────────────────────────┐
            │  1. Enter or Edit data                        │
            │  2. Create new data file from .QES file       │
            │                                               │
            │  3. Revise structure of data file using revised .QES │
            │     Note: uses current century converting YY -> YYYY! │
            │  4. Reenter and verify records in existing data file │
            │  5. Rebuild index file(s) specified in .CHK file │
            └──────────────────────────────────────────────┘



                         Choose one: 1


                  The default path is C:\EPI6

                           OK   N


      F2-Setup                      F9-List files     F10-Done
```

The ENTER program can save each file with the same filename as you created in EPED, but suffixed with **.REC**. This suffix is automatically added by the program when you convert your .QES file to data entry format.

Opening .REC files

To open files in the ENTER program, follow these steps:

1 Highlight ENTER from the PROGRAMS menu and press ⟨ENTER⟩.
2 Type the name of the .REC file you wish to open (press **F9** for a list of files if you cannot remember the filename) and press ⟨ENTER⟩.
3 Type 1, and press ⟨ENTER⟩.
4 Press ⟨ENTER⟩ again to confirm.

Problems opening .REC files

In certain versions of Windows, you may see a message saying that a .REC file cannot be opened, because it is a 'Read-Only' file. This may happen if you have copied a .REC file over from a CD-ROM. In this situation, the following should solve the problem (you will only have to do this once for each .REC file):

1 Press **F10** to clear the message, and again to leave the ENTER program.
2 Open Windows Explorer, and click on the EPI6 folder.
3 Find and click the right-hand mouse button on the .REC file concerned.
4 Click on PROPERTIES – under 'Attributes', the box marked 'Read-Only' will be checked.
5 Click the box to uncheck 'Read-Only'.
6 Click 'Apply'.
7 Click 'OK'.
8 Close Windows Explorer.
9 Open Epi Info, and open the ENTER program.
10 Open the .REC file and enter data (described below).

Entering data

To enter data, type information into the boxes that appear after each field name. If you fill a field with text, the cursor automatically moves on to the next field. Otherwise, pressing ⟨**ENTER**⟩ will move you to the next field. If you accidentally go too far, and advance by two fields, just press the 'up arrow' (↑) key until you are on the correct field again. A 'beep' sounds if you make an entry error.

Some fields only accept certain kinds of data. The prompt line, near the bottom of the screen, displays what type of data can be entered (e.g. Y or N only, numbers only, text or specific words only). On certain fields, a menu of available choices can be viewed by pressing **F9**.

Note: you do *not* have to enter all of the data at once! You can exit from the program after inputting some data then go back in at a later date to add more. When re-entering a .REC file, you will be presented with the next available record number in the sequence.

Moving around the data entry screen

The following keys can help you to move around while entering information:

- Up or down arrow keys – move the cursor to the previous or next field.
- Right or left arrow keys – move the cursor one space right or left.
- **Home** moves the cursor to the first field in the record.
- **End** goes to the end of the record.
- **Del** deletes the last character entered.
- **Page Up** or **Page Down** moves up or down a whole page.

Saving information

When you have filled in all of the fields for a particular record, the following message is displayed:

```
'Write data to disk? (Y/N)'
```

Type **Y** if you wish to save the record, or **N** to discard it.

Moving between records

ENTER automatically assigns an incremental number to each record, starting with the first one entered. The record number appears in the lower right-hand corner of the screen. It is possible to move (or browse) between records by pressing **F7** (backwards) or **F8** (forwards).

Searching for specific records

By pressing **Ctrl** and F simultaneously, you can find a particular record, by specifying either its record number or another field. For example, you could find a specific patient identifier thus:

1 Access the ENTER program.
2 Open the file concerned (*see* p. 56).
3 Press **Ctrl** and F simultaneously.
4 Type the required name* into the 'ID' field (or into the appropriate field in *your* database).
5 Press **F3**.
6 Any records with matching names (if any exist) then appear.
7 Select the required record using the arrow keys, and press ⟨ENTER⟩.

If you cannot remember exactly what the name is, or how it is spelt, type in as much as you can, followed by an asterisk. So if the name you wanted was '00461', you could type 004, and every identifier starting with '004' would be then displayed.

In step 4 above, you can enter 'search' information for more than one field. If, for instance, you wish to find records of people with diagnosed hypertension who are also aged 33:

1 Enter Y in your hypertension field (assuming it is in this format).
2 In the 'AGE' field, type 33.
3 Press **F3**.

If any records match those criteria, they are displayed. Otherwise, you will see a message:

```
Record not found. Press Esc
```

If you wish to find a particular record by its *record number*:

1 Access the ENTER program.
2 Open the file concerned.
3 Press **Ctrl** and F simultaneously.
4 Press **F2**.
5 Enter the record number required.
6 Press ⟨ENTER⟩.

If it exists, the record is displayed.

Editing data already entered

The data in records can still be edited, even after they have been saved.

1 Using the procedures outlined above in 'Moving between records' and 'Searching for specific records', display the particular record that you wish to edit.
2 Make changes to the required fields.
3 Press the **End** key.

4 Save the record, if you are happy with it, by pressing Y.

5 Exit the program by pressing **F10**, or select another record to edit.

Note: changes must be saved before you move to another record, or they will be ignored and the edited record will return to its previous state.

Deleting and undeleting records

When a record is displayed on the screen, pressing **F6** marks it as deleted, and an asterisk is placed against the record number. Deleted records can be made active again by pressing **F6** once more.

If you mark a record as deleted, its data remain visible on screen, but are not included in any analysis carried out on the file concerned.

Printing records

A print can be made of any or all of the records in a particular file by pressing **F5** and following instructions on-screen. You can produce a 'master printout' of the questionnaire/form (which can be copied and used as a proforma) by printing the form before you begin inputting data. This has lines printed next to all the field names, suitable for making manual entries.

Exiting the ENTER program

Press **F10** to exit the ENTER program, and return to the EPI6 menu.

ANALYSIS

When ANALYSIS is accessed through the PROGRAMS menu, this screen will appear:

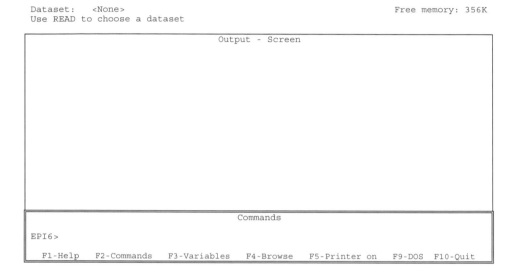

```
Dataset:    <None>                                    Free memory: 356K
Use READ to choose a dataset
```

Analysing data

To analyse data:

- Access the appropriate file.
- For each field you want to analyse, enter a **command**, specifying what form you would like the analysis presented in, e.g. table, list, pie or bar-chart.
- Then specify a **variable** (field name), e.g. name, age, occupation.

Follow these steps:

1 At the EPI6> prompt, type read.
2 Press ⟨ENTER⟩.
3 Select a file from the menu which will appear at the top of the screen.
4 Press ⟨ENTER⟩.
5 Decide whether you would like the information displayed on the screen or printed out. Information will default to the screen – pressing **F5** routes to the printer; pressing it again routes back to the screen.
6 Press **F2** to select a command.
7 Press **F3** to choose a variable.
8 Press ⟨ENTER⟩.

Press **Esc** to remove any menus you have called up, if they are not required.

Commands

These are some of the commands available – you can either type them in at the EPI> prompt or press **F2** for a full listing, which can then be selected using the arrow keys.

- **LIST** – produces a listing of any field.
- **FREQ** – counts categories in a particular variable. It produces a table showing how often each category is recorded and percentages (e.g. if 'sex' was a variable, it would state how many males and how many females were recorded).
- **TABLES** – produces a table for one or more variables at the same time (e.g. name age would show all individuals' names, with their ages displayed at the side). Where appropriate, this command also calculates measures of association such as the chi-squared test, relative risk and odds ratio.
- **GRAPHS** and **CHARTS** – the following are available: pie, bar, histogram, scatter, line. While the graphs produced are reasonably clear, they are not a major strongpoint of Epi Info (a couple of examples are shown in Chapter 10). There is very little flexibility in controlling their appearance, and they cannot be transferred into a word processing application such as Word, for incorporation into a report or other document. *See* p. 85 for some suggestions on how to overcome this problem.
- **TITLES** – allows you to add up to five lines of text, which appear at the top of a table, frequency, chart or graph. At the EPI> prompt, you could, for example, type:

TITLE 1 Audit of patients in Bromfield Surgery
TITLE 2 by Audrey Spencer

Note: always leave a space between 'TITLE' and the number. Then analyse as normal (e.g. PIE GENDER) – the title(s) will be displayed. To remove the titles, type: **TITLE 1** and ⟨ENTER⟩ – this removes all titles with numbers 1 or greater.

- **BROWSE** – pressing **F4** allows you to browse through all of the data in a file, displayed in tabular (or spreadsheet) form.
- **UPDATE** – this is similar to the BROWSE command, except that it allows you to edit data which have already been entered, saving you the trouble of having to leave ANALYSIS and go into ENTER. After making each change, press ⟨ENTER⟩. You will automatically be prompted to

save the change, or cancel it. When you have finished editing, press **F10** to exit UPDATE. *Caution*: Any changes you make within UPDATE will be permanent – be absolutely sure of your actions before saving them, and create a backup copy of your file first.

- **SORT** – puts records into a particular order. If the field holds names, they are sorted into alphabetical order; if numbers are recorded, they are sorted into number order (e.g. sort name or sort age). You can sort more than one field at a time (e.g. sort name age). To clear a sort operation, type SORT without any other instructions.
- **SELECT** – allows you to work with a subset of the data in a file. This lets you analyse information only for various categories within variables. For example, if you wish to select only females less than 40 years old, type:

1 SELECT SEX = "F"
2 Press ⟨ENTER⟩
3 SELECT AGE < 40
4 Press ⟨ENTER⟩

or you could select only females aged over 20 and under 40:

1 SELECT SEX = "F"
2 Press ⟨ENTER⟩
3 SELECT AGE > 20
4 Press ⟨ENTER⟩
5 SELECT AGE < 40
6 Press ⟨ENTER⟩

The following operators can be used:

Operator	Meaning	Example	Selects
>	Greater than	select height > 1.5	all heights over 1.5 m
<	Less than	select age < 35	all ages below 35
=	Equal to	select sex = "F"	all females
<=	Less than or equal to	select age <= 35	all ages 35 or under
>=	Greater than or equal to	select age >= 35	all ages 35 or over
<>	Not equal to	select age <> 35	all ages except 35
AND	logical 'AND'	select sex = "F" and age < 35	all females aged under 35
OR	logical 'OR'	select job = "NURSE" or job = "PHYSIO"	all nurses *or* physiotherapists

Both numeric and alphanumeric variables can be used with the above commands. For example, you can select only surnames which begin with letters between H and S by typing:

SELECT SURNAME > "H" AND SURNAME < "S"

Performing a

```
LIST SURNAME
```

will not display surnames beginning with A, B, C, D, E, F, G, H, S, T, U, V, W, X, Y or Z. You should enclose character values (e.g. "H") in double quotes. Do *not* use double quotes for numeric values, though.

To clear a selection operation, simply type SELECT without any other instructions and press ⟨ENTER⟩.

To change a selection operation, first clear the selection criteria by using the SELECT command on its own. The SELECT command is incremental, so if you do not clear the old selection, it will simply be added to the existing criteria using the AND operator and give incorrect analysis results.

The current selection criteria are shown at the top of the screen, and printed above each list and table that ANALYSIS produces.

Variables

These are your field names, created at the EPED stage. You can either type them in after a command at the EPI> prompt, or press **F3** to see a listing of all the variables available, which can be selected using the arrow keys.

More than one variable can be specified, so you could, for instance, type:

```
LIST NAME OCCUPATION
```

This would give you a listing of all individuals' names, and *also* their occupations, in the same analysis.

If you wish to select multiple variables using the **F3** menu:

1 Type in a command (e.g. **List** or **Tables**).
2 Press **F3**.
3 Highlight a variable (using the arrow keys).
4 Press **Shift** and + simultaneously. The variable will now be marked with a '▶'.
5 Repeat steps 3 and 4 for each variable needed.
6 Press ⟨ENTER⟩ when all are marked. Every variable marked will have been placed after the command you specified.
7 Press ⟨ENTER⟩ again to perform the analysis.

Printing in ANALYSIS

In this program, pressing **F5** 'toggles' (switches alternately) between outputting information to the screen or the printer *and* screen. When you enter ANALYSIS, information automatically goes to the screen. To print an analysis (e.g. a listing of AGE):

1 Press **F5**.
2 **LIST AGE**.
3 Press ⟨ENTER⟩.

This should now print. To switch back from printer output to screen output only, or vice versa, press **F5**. Refer to p. 82 if you have any problems with printing in Epi Info.

Exiting ANALYSIS

Press **F10** to return to the EPI menu.

5

Basic tutorial exercises in Epi Info

Patient satisfaction audit

Introduction

In this exercise we will work through the steps required to enter and analyse data from a patient satisfaction survey. It is worth spending a little time working through the exercise as you will gain some valuable 'hands-on' experience of using Epi Info.

Background

The St Elsewhere's GUM clinic is a busy urban genito-urinary medicine clinic seeing between 15 000 and 18 000 patients per year. The clinic operates a mixed appointments and walk-in service at the following times:

Day	Times	Notes
Monday	09.00–11.15	Same-day HIV testing by appointment
	13.00–17.45	
Tuesday	14.00–16.15	Morning HIV appointments only
Wednesday	09.30–11.45	
	14.00–16.15	
Thursday	14.00–17.45	Morning appointments only
Friday	09.30–11.45	
	14.00–16.15	

All sessions are mixed sex with separate-sex waiting rooms and access to clinical areas.

St Elsewhere's is a large and modern teaching hospital, but the GUM clinic is in Portakabin accommodation on an older part of the hospital site. The clinic hopes to receive funds to relocate to purpose-built accommodation within the next two years.

Aims

The audit aims to improve the service at a GUM clinic. This will be done by assessing patient satisfaction with various aspects of the services provided and, by analysis of responses, considering whether any improvements should be made.

Criteria and standards

At least 90% of patients should be satisfied or very satisfied with the following aspects of the service:

- reading material in waiting rooms
- information displayed in waiting rooms
- condition of the waiting rooms
- overall service received
- their welcome on arrival
- medical treatment received
- nursing treatment
- health advice received
- information about diagnosis.

At least 80% of patients should state that they would recommend the clinic to a friend. This is set lower, as some people would not admit the attendance of a GUM clinic that the criterion assumes.

Methodology

For a period of one week every patient attending the clinic will be asked to fill in a short questionnaire and return it to reception before leaving. The data will be entered into Epi Info and results produced. These will be compared with the standards already set, and conclusions will be drawn as to whether any improvements should be made. A poster summarising the results of the audit and any changes made as a result of it will be displayed in the waiting rooms for patients to see. The audit will be repeated in 12 months to re-evaluate patient satisfaction and assess whether changes have been effective.

The data collection form

The data collection form used to collect the data for the patient satisfaction audit is shown on the following pages.

ST ELSEWHERE'S GUM CLINIC
PATIENT SATISFACTION SURVEY

We are asking patients how satisfied they are with services in this clinic so that we can make improvements to the service. Please can you help us by completing this questionnaire. Your answers will be **completely confidential** and will not be seen by staff at the clinic.

How to fill in the questionnaire:

Most of the questions ask how satisfied you are with different aspects of the facilities and services at this clinic. Look for the box which is closest to your own view, and mark with a tick as shown:

(If there are any questions which you think do not apply to you, please leave these blank.)

The following guide will help you decide how to answer.

☺ If you are completely happy with a particular aspect of the service, tick the box under 'very satisfied'.

☺ If you are basically happy with a particular aspect of the service and do not have any major concerns, tick the box under 'satisfied'.

☺ If you have some concerns about a particular aspect of the service and are not completely satisfied, tick the box under 'dissatisfied'.

☹ If you are very unhappy with a particular aspect of the service, tick the box under 'very dissatisfied'.

What do you think about the following:

Please answer the following questions about the service you have received today:

1 Facilities at this clinic

	very satisfied ☺	satisfied ☺	dissatisfied ☺	very dissatisfied ☹
(a) Reading material in the waiting room (e.g. magazines)	1 ☐	2 ☐	3 ☐	4 ☐
(b) The information displayed in this clinic (notices, health education leaflets, etc.)	1 ☐	2 ☐	3 ☐	4 ☐
(c) Waiting room (chairs, carpeting and decorating, etc.)	1 ☐	2 ☐	3 ☐	4 ☐

PLEASE CONTINUE

2 Your treatment at this clinic
(Leave blank if you have not had any of the treatments mentioned below)

	very satisfied ☺	satisfied ☺	dissatisfied ☺	very dissatisfied ☹
(a) The overall service at the clinic	1 ☐	2 ☐	3 ☐	4 ☐
(b) The welcome on arrival at reception	1 ☐	2 ☐	3 ☐	4 ☐
(c) The medical treatment you received today	1 ☐	2 ☐	3 ☐	4 ☐
(d) The nursing treatment you received today	1 ☐	2 ☐	3 ☐	4 ☐
(e) The health advice you received today	1 ☐	2 ☐	3 ☐	4 ☐
(f) The information given to you about your diagnosis/condition	1 ☐	2 ☐	3 ☐	4 ☐

3 Which waiting system would you prefer?
(a) An appointment system, where you may have to wait several days for   a ☐
an appointment, but will have a specific time to attend the clinic.
(b) A non-appointment system, where you are seen on a first-come,   b ☐
first-served basis. (You can walk in when you want, but may have
to wait up to an hour or more to be seen.)

4 What would be the most useful opening times for this clinic?

Early morning (8–9 am)	1 ☐ Yes	2 ☐ No
Morning (from 9 am)	1 ☐ Yes	2 ☐ No
Lunchtime (12–2pm)	1 ☐ Yes	2 ☐ No
Afternoon (up to 5 pm)	1 ☐ Yes	2 ☐ No
Evening (up to 7.30 pm)	1 ☐ Yes	2 ☐ No

5 Would you prefer to visit a clinic which is specifically for a particular group, e.g. women
only, men only, gay men, young people?

     1 ☐ Yes   2 ☐ No

If **yes,** please specify what type of clinic you would like to attend:

6 Would you recommend this clinic to a friend?

     1 ☐ Yes   2 ☐ No

Why?

7 What is your gender?

     1 ☐ Male   2 ☐ Female

How old are you? _____

Which of the following do you consider best describes your ethnic origin? (Please tick
the relevant box)

1 ☐ White	2 ☐ Black African	3 ☐ Black Caribbean
4 ☐ Black Other	5 ☐ Indian	6 ☐ Bangladeshi
7 ☐ Pakistani	8 ☐ Chinese	9 ☐ Other

Thank you for taking the time to complete this questionnaire

Setting up the data-entry screens

Start EPED and type the following questionnaire:

```
St Elsewhere's GUM Clinic – Patient Satisfaction Survey
1 Facilities at this clinic
     {Reading} material                                    #
     Information {Display}ed                               #
     Waiting {Room}                                        #


2 Your treatment at this clinic
     Overall {Service}                                     #
     {Welcome} on arrival                                  #
     {Medical} treatment                                   #
     {Nursing} treatment                                   #
     Health {advice}                                       #
     {Info}rmation                                         #


3 Which {waiting} system do you prefer?                    #


4 When you visit this clinic which times would you
  prefer:
     {Early}                                               #
     {Morning}                                             #
     {Lunch}                                               #
     {Afternoon}                                           #
     {Evening}                                             #


5 Would you {prefer} to visit a clinic . . .               #
  If YES, what type of {clinic}?                           #


6 Would you recommend this clinic to a {friend}?  #
  Why?  〈AAAAAAAAAAAAAAAAAAAAAAAAAAAAAAAAAAAAAAAA〉


7 {Sex}                                                    #
  {Age}                                                    #
  {Ethnic} Group:                                          #
```

Save the questionnaire (**F9**) as GUMSAT.QES. Note the names (enclosed by { } characters), lengths and types given to the variables.

Creating the data-entry system

Start ENTER and specify the following.

Prompt	You type	Meaning
Data file (.REC):	GUMSAT	Name of data file to be created
Choose one:	2	Create new data file from .QES file
New Questionnaire file (.QES):	GUMSAT	Template used to create file
OK:	Y	Everything is OK

The screen should look like this:

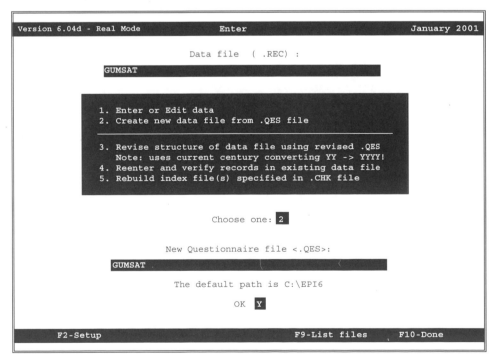

Press **F4** to create the new data file (GUMSAT.REC). The data entry screen appears. Do *not* enter any data now. Instead, press **F10** to quit.

Setting up checks

You *could* start entering data straight away, but it is better to set up some checks that will ensure that fewer errors occur in your data. Start CHECK and specify GUMSAT to the 'Data file (.REC):' prompt and press the ⟨ENTER⟩ key. Use the function keys to set up the following checks:

Variable	Checks	You type (in the relevant field)	
reading	Legal values 1, 2, 3, 4	1 ⟨F1⟩	4 ⟨F2⟩
display	Legal values 1, 2, 3, 4	1 ⟨F1⟩	4 ⟨F2⟩
room	Legal values 1, 2, 3, 4	1 ⟨F1⟩	4 ⟨F2⟩
service	Legal values 1, 2, 3, 4	1 ⟨F1⟩	4 ⟨F2⟩
welcome	Legal values 1, 2, 3, 4	1 ⟨F1⟩	4 ⟨F2⟩
medical	Legal values 1, 2, 3, 4	1 ⟨F1⟩	4 ⟨F2⟩
nursing	Legal values 1, 2, 3, 4	1 ⟨F1⟩	4 ⟨F2⟩
advice	Legal values 1, 2, 3, 4	1 ⟨F1⟩	4 ⟨F2⟩
info	Legal values 1, 2, 3, 4	1 ⟨F1⟩	4 ⟨F2⟩
waiting	Legal values 1, 2, 3, 4	1 ⟨F1⟩	4 ⟨F2⟩
early	Legal values 1, 2	1 ⟨F6⟩	4 ⟨F6⟩
morning	Legal values 1, 2	1 ⟨F6⟩	4 ⟨F6⟩
lunch	Legal values 1, 2	1 ⟨F6⟩	2 ⟨F6⟩
afternoon	Legal values 1, 2	1 ⟨F6⟩	2 ⟨F6⟩
evening	Legal values 1, 2	1 ⟨F6⟩	2 ⟨F6⟩
prefer	Legal values 1, 2	1 ⟨F6⟩	2 ⟨F6⟩
	Jump on '2' to friend	2 ⟨F7⟩ – move to friend ⟨F7⟩	
clinic	Legal values 1, 2, 3, 4	1 ⟨F1⟩	4 ⟨F2⟩
friend	Legal values 1, 2	1 ⟨F6⟩	2 ⟨F6⟩
sex	Legal values 1, 2	1 ⟨F6⟩	2 ⟨F6⟩
age	Range 14 to 85	14 ⟨F1⟩	85 ⟨F2⟩
ethnic	Range 1 to 9	1 ⟨F1⟩	9 ⟨F2⟩

Press **F10** and answer 'Y' to the 'Write data to disk [Y/N/Esc]?' prompt. Now start ENTER and enter some data into the GUMSAT data file. Make sure the data-entry checks are working correctly. Press **F10** to quit.

Beware: the CHECK screen looks very like the data-entry screen. Do not confuse the two.

Sample analysis

The real data from this audit is stored in the file PATSAT.REC (you should have already copied this file over from your CD-ROM to the EPI6 directory – if you have not done this, refer to p. 46, 'Copying the example Epi Info files'). Start ANALYSIS and open the file PATSAT.REC by typing:

```
READ PATSAT.REC
```

Press ⟨ENTER⟩. *Note*: if you have difficulties working with this file, it may be stored as a 'Read-Only' file. To correct this, please see instructions on p. 56.

You can examine this dataset (in spreadsheet format) by typing:

```
BROWSE
```

Press ⟨ENTER⟩. Press **F4** to see individual records displayed full screen. Use the up and down arrow keys to move between variables, noting the names of the variables and their meaning:

Variable	Description	Codes
reading	Level of satisfaction with reading material in waiting room	1 = Very satisfied 2 = Satisfied 3 = Dissatisfied 4 = Very Dissatisfied
display	Level of satisfaction with information display	As ready (above)
room	Level of satisfaction with the waiting room	As reading (above)
service	Level of satisfaction with overall service	As reading (above)
welcome	Level of satisfaction with welcome	As reading (above)
medical	Level of satisfaction with medical treatment	As reading (above)
nursing	Level of satisfaction with nursing treatment	As reading (above)
advice	Level of satisfaction with health advice	As reading (above)
info	Level of satisfaction with information about diagnosis	As reading (above)
waiting	Preferred waiting system	1 = Appointment 2 = Walk-in
early	Useful opening time EARLY MORNING	1 = Yes, 2 = No
morning	Useful opening time MORNING	As early (above)
lunch	Useful opening time LUNCH	As early (above)
afternoon	Useful opening time AFTERNOON	As early (above)
evening	Useful opening time EVENING	As early (above)
prefer	Prefer to visit a specialist clinic	As early (above)

Continued

Variable	Description	Codes
clinic	Type of clinic preferred	1 = Gay men
		2 = Women only
		3 = Men only
		4 = Young people
friend	Recommend clinic to a friend	1 = Yes, 2 = No
sex	Sex	1 = Male,
		2 = Female
age	Age	14–85
ethnic	Ethnic group	1 = White
		2 = Black African
		3 = Black Caribbean
		4 = Black Other
		5 = Indian
		6 = Bangladeshi
		7 = Pakistani
		8 = Chinese
		9 = Other

Examine the frequency distribution of the READING variable with the FREQ command:

```
FREQ READING
```
Press ⟨ENTER⟩

which produces the following output:

```
READING | Freq      Percent      Cum.
--------+---------------------------------
1       |    21      14.6%        14.6%
2       |    72      50.0%        64.6%
3       |    38      26.4%        91.0%
4       |    13       9.0%       100.0%
--------+---------------------------------
Total   |   144     100.0%
```

Ignore the statistics under the tables as they mean nothing in this context. Instead, examine the table closely. Only 64.6% of respondents (14.6% + 50.0% = 64.6%) said they were happy with the reading material in the waiting rooms:

```
READING | Freq     Percent     Cum.
--------+---------------------------
   1    |    21     14.6%       14.6%
   2    |    72     50.0%       64.6%
   3    |    38     26.4%       91.0%
   4    |    13      9.0%      100.0%
--------+---------------------------
 Total  |   144    100.0%
```

Use the FREQ command to examine the distributions of the other satisfaction variables. The following table summarises the levels of satisfaction found:

Variable	Result	Standard
reading	64.6%	90.0%
display	98.6%	90.0%
room	96.6%	90.0%
service	98.2%	90.0%
welcome	95.6%	90.0%
medical	99.0%	90.0%
nursing	97.0%	90.0%
advice	98.0%	90.0%
info	94.0%	90.0%
friend	94.4%	80.0%

The clinic met all its targets except for the quality of reading material provided in the waiting rooms.

You can examine the data further using the TABLES command:

TABLES SEX READING

Press ⟨ENTER⟩. If you examine the resulting table carefully you may see that there is some difference in the distribution of the READING variables between males (1) and females (2):

```
                        READING
SEX      |    1      2      3      4  | Total
---------+---------------------------+------
    1    |    5     20     16      9  |    50
    2    |   16     44     19      4  |    83
---------+---------------------------+------
 Total   |   21     64     35     13  |   133
```

You can see this clearly if you look at the row percentages in the table by issuing the following commands:

```
SET PERCENTS = ON
Press ⟨ENTER⟩
TABLES SEX READING
Press ⟨ENTER⟩
```

which produces the following output:

```
                              READING
 SEX        |      1        2        3        4 |  Total
 -----------+----------------------------------+-------
        1   |      5       20       16        9 |     50
            >  10.0%    40.0%    32.0%    18.0% >  37.6%
            |  23.8%    31.3%    45.7%    69.2% |
        2   |     16       44       19        4 |     83
            >  19.3%    53.0%    22.9%     4.8% >  62.4%
            |  76.2%    68.8%    54.3%    30.8% |
 -----------+----------------------------------+-------
    Total   |     21       64       35       13 |    133
            |  15.8%    48.1%    26.3%     9.8% |
```

The females were more likely to report being very satisfied or satisfied (19.3% + 53.0% = 72.3%) than the males (10.0% + 40.0% = 50.0%).

Use the TABLES command to check for any other male/female differences in the data. You can use the same commands to examine the other variables collected in the audit. For example, the command:

```
FREQ WAITING
Press ⟨ENTER⟩
```

shows that the current mixed appointment (1) and walk-in (2) system suits the clinic's clients:

```
 WAITING  |  Freq    Percent     Cum.
 ---------+-----------------------------
 1        |    25    18.4%      18.4%
 2        |   111    81.6%     100.0%
 ---------+-----------------------------
    Total |   136   100.0%
```

Use the FREQ command to examine the 'useful opening times' variables (EARLY, MORNING, LUNCH, AFTERNOON and EVENING). Are the current clinic opening times meeting their clients' needs?

Examine the PREFER and CLINIC variables. Is the current mixed-sex clinic format suitable?

Some advanced analysis features of Epi Info

Converting dates of birth into age values

In ANALYSIS with a dataset selected, type:

1 DEFINE AGE # # #
2 Press ⟨ENTER⟩
3 LET AGE = ("06/08/2003" − DOB) DIV 365.25
4 Press ⟨ENTER⟩
5 FREQ AGE
6 Press ⟨ENTER⟩

This assumes the following about your file:

- The fieldname for the *date of birth* field is 'DOB'.
- The *date of birth* field is in DD/MM/YYYY format.
- Today's date is 06/08/2003 (and that you want to calculate the age from this date. You may, for instance, want to calculate the age from the date of the original survey − in this case, enter the date required).

Creating age bands

In ANALYSIS (with a dataset selected), type:

1 DEFINE AGEGROUP ⟨AAAAAAAAAAAA⟩
2 Press ⟨ENTER⟩
3 RECODE AGE (or name of age field) TO AGEGROUP 15-24 = "15-24"
   25-34 = "25-34" . . . . **etc.**
4 Press ⟨ENTER⟩
5 FREQ AGEGROUP
6 Press ⟨ENTER⟩

Calculating BMI

This can be useful if you have details of patients' height and weight, but do not already have a BMI value recorded.

In ANALYSIS (with a dataset selected), type:

1 DEFINE BMI # # . #
2 Press ⟨ENTER⟩
3 LET BMI = WEIGHT/(HEIGHT^2)
4 Press ⟨ENTER⟩
5 FREQ BMI
6 Press ⟨ENTER⟩

This assumes that:

• your file contains the fieldnames 'height' and 'weight'
• height is in metres
• weight is in kilograms.

If this is *not* the case, substitute one of the following commands:

Weight	Height	Command
pounds	inches	let bmi = (weight/2.205)/((height * 0.0254)^2)
kilograms	inches	let bmi = weight/((height * 0.0254) ^2)
pounds	metres	let bmi = (weight/2.205)/(height^2)
stones	feet	let bmi = (weight * 6.305)/((height * 0.3048)^2)

The IF . . . THEN command

This command allows you to analyse a value of a variable if certain condition(s) are met. For example, people whose BMI is over 30 are usually regarded as being *obese*, those with a BMI of more than 25 to 30 are *overweight*, while those with a BMI of under 19 are usually regarded as being *underweight*. Anyone whose BMI is between 19 and 25 could be classed as *normal*. Epi Info can be instructed to automatically look at every BMI value and analyse the words 'obese', 'overweight', 'normal', 'underweight' or any others, depending on the BMI value.

Assuming that you have a field called BMI in your database, at the EPI6> prompt within ANALYSIS, type:

1 `DEFINE BMIGROUP ⟨AAAAAAAAAAAAAAA⟩`
2 Press ⟨ENTER⟩
3 `IF BMI <19 THEN BMIGROUP="UNDERWEIGHT"`
4 Press ⟨ENTER⟩
5 `IF BMI >=19 AND <=25 THEN BMIGROUP="NORMAL"`
6 Press ⟨ENTER⟩
7 `IF BMI >25 AND <=30 THEN BMIGROUP="OVERWEIGHT"`
8 Press ⟨ENTER⟩
9 `IF BMI >30 THEN BMIGROUP="OBESE"`
10 Press ⟨ENTER⟩
11 `FREQ BMIGROUP`
12 Press ⟨ENTER⟩

The DEFINE command creates a new text field called BMIGROUP which is 15 characters long.

The first IF . . . THEN command tells ANALYSIS that if the number in the BMI field is less than 19, then the description 'underweight' will be analysed by the new field.

The second IF . . . THEN command tells ANALYSIS that if the number in the BMI field is greater than or equal to 19 AND less than or equal to 25, then the description 'normal' will be analysed by the new field.

The third IF . . . THEN command tells ANALYSIS that if the number in the BMI field is greater than 25 and less than or equal to 30, then the description 'overweight' will be inserted into the new field.

The final IF . . . THEN command tells ANALYSIS that if the number in the BMI field is greater than 30, then the description 'obese' will be inserted into the new field.

The FREQ command produces a frequency table, indicating how many people on the database are 'obese', 'overweight', 'normal' or 'underweight'.

Note: the above example assumes that the fieldnames containing people's heights and weights are called HEIGHT and WEIGHT. If this is not the case, substitute the field names of your height and weight fields.

If you type

`LIST BMI BMIGROUP`

and press ⟨ENTER⟩, each individual BMI will be listed, together with a description of either 'obese', 'overweight', 'normal' or 'underweight' by its side.

Operators for calculated fields

You may have noticed that the LET command discussed previously contains instructions telling the program to transform existing data into new data, using ranges of values or calculations. The most common operators for these calculations are:

+	Addition
−	Subtraction
*	Multiplication
/	Division
DIV	Division and rounding *down* the result (i.e. discarding the remainder) to return to a whole number result
^2	Squared
^0.5	Square root
^	Exponent – raises a number by the power indicated
(	Used for grouping within an expression[†]
)	Used for grouping within an expression[†]
>	Greater than*
<	Less than*
>=	Greater than or equal to*
<=	Less than or equal to*
=	Equal to*
<>	Not equal to*
[	Beginning of substring[‡]
]	End of substring[‡]
TRUNC (x)	Rounds *down* to the nearest whole number
ROUND (x)	Rounds *up* to the nearest whole number, if the fraction is 0.5 or more
AND	If everything being **AND**ed is true, then the expression is true*
OR	If one or more (i.e. any) of the conditions being **OR**ed are true, then the expression is true*

[†] An expression is a combination of variables, values and operators which can be evaluated to produce a single result (e.g. let bmi = weight/height^2). The order in which calculations are made within an expression follows the BEDMAS order (**B**rackets, **E**xponent, **D**ivision, **M**ultiplication, **A**ddition, **S**ubtraction). Expressions in brackets or with exponent functions are evaluated first, followed by multiplication and division, followed by addition and subtraction.
* These operators are only used with IF, THEN and SELECT commands.
[‡] Substring operators work with character and date type variables, and require you to specify a starting position and a length. For example, if the variable DATE contains the data '20/10/61' then the command let month = date[4,2] would extract the month '10' from the DATE variable.

Some other ANALYSIS commands

- SET PAUSE = ON
  Prevents data scrolling down the screen before you can read it. This command allows you to scroll slowly using the ⟨ENTER⟩ key. Use SET PAUSE = OFF to discontinue this.
- SET PERCENTS = ON
  Tables will be displayed with percentages below each count. Row percentages are printed first, with an arrow pointing to the denominator on the right. Column percentages are printed below the row percentages. Use SET PERCENTS = OFF to turn the percentages off.
- SET LINES = ON
  Tables will be displayed with lines separating each cell. This can aid the ease of reading and interpretation. Use SET LINES = OFF to eradicate the lines.
- SET STATISTICS = OFF
  Prevents statistics being produced for each table. Use SET STATISTICS = ON to reactivate the statistics.
- SET PRINTER = EPSON   (Epson/IBM dot matrix)
                LQ1500   (Epson LQ1500)
                HP   (HP Laser)
                PLOTTER
                HP7475   (Plotter)
                HP7550   (Plotter)
  set pmode = 5   (5,4,3,2,1 or 0)   5 is highest quality and full page.

Saving SET commands

This allows you to place any SET commands you like into a file called CONFIG.EPI. This file automatically loads and runs these commands every time you start ANALYSIS. It is especially useful for commands such as SET PRINTER as you will probably want to specify the same printer driver all the time. Storing commands in a CONFIG.EPI file saves you the trouble of typing the command every time you use ANALYSIS. It is a special program file that runs automatically whenever ANALYSIS is started.

To set up a CONFIG.EPI file:

1 In ANALYSIS type: EDIT CONFIG.EPI
2 Press ⟨ENTER⟩

3 Type: SET PRINTER = $LJ (assuming that you have an HP laserjet printer)
4 Press **F2** – this saves the file
5 Press **F10** – this exits back into ANALYSIS

Your printer driver is now set. Note that the changes will not take effect until you quit and restart ANALYSIS. The above steps work with any SET command – just type the SET command you require in step 3, above.

To add, remove or edit SET commands:

1 In ANALYSIS type: EDIT CONFIG.EPI
2 Press ⟨ENTER⟩
3 Use the arrow, ⟨ENTER⟩ and **Backspace** keys to locate and edit commands as necessary
4 Press **F2** – this saves the file
5 Press **F10** – this exits back into ANALYSIS

A typical CONFIG.EPI file might look like this:

```
SET PRINTER = $LJ
SET PMODE = 5
SET PAUSE = ON
SET PAGE = 72,88
```

Saving an analysis

If you need to perform certain ANALYSIS commands on a number of occasions, a series of commands can be saved in a program (.PGM) file.

After performing a set of analyses, type:

SAVE (filename) .PGM (e.g. SAVE DIABETES.PGM)

Press ⟨ENTER⟩.

To run the saved analysis programme, in ANALYSIS, select required dataset and press ⟨ENTER⟩. Type:

RUN (filename) .PGM (e.g. RUN DIABETES.PGM)

Press ⟨ENTER⟩ again. The analysis program will now run. Press **Page Up** or **Page Down** as required, to scroll through the analysis.

Solving printing problems

While Epi Info normally prints text and tables without too much difficulty, graphics tend to present problems. If you find that Epi Info will not print something, the following procedures will hopefully do the trick.

Install a printer driver

ANALYSIS normally outputs for a text printer, but you can select others by using the SET PRINTER command. At the EPI6> prompt in ANALYSIS, type:

SET PRINTER = ⟨driver name⟩ ⟨ENTER⟩ (e.g. SET PRINTER = $LJ3R)

Available drivers are:

$FX	Epson FX80 printer
$PS	Postscript printers
$CFX	Epson 9-pin colour printer
$CLQ	Epson 24-pin colour printer
$DJ	Hewlett-Packard deskjet
$DJC	Hewlett-Packard colour deskjet
$HP7090	HP Plotter 7090
$HP7470	HP Plotter 7470
$HP7475	HP Plotter 7475
$HP7550	HP Plotter 7550
$HP7585	HP Plotter 7585
$HP7595	HP Plotter 7595
$IBMQ	IBM Quietwriter printer
$LJ	Hewlett-Packard laserjet
$LJ3R	Hewlett-Packard laserjet III
$LQ	Epson 24-pin printer
$OKI92	Okidata 92 printer
$PJ	Hewlett-Packard paintjet printer
$PP24	IBM Proprinter, 24 pin
$TSH	Toshiba 24-pin printer

If your printer is not on the above list, consult your printer's user manual to see if your printer can emulate any of the above. If so, set your printer up for the most suitable emulation and use the appropriate SET PRINTER driver.

If you have a dot-matrix printer, try either:

SET PRINTER = $FX   or   SET PRINTER = $LQ

If you have an inkjet printer, try either:

SET PRINTER = $DJ   or   SET PRINTER = DJC

If you have a laser printer, try either:

SET PRINTER = $LJ   or   SET PRINTER = $PS (if Postscript)

You can set up the SET PRINTER command so that it automatically loads every time you use ANALYSIS. See p. 81 'Saving SET commands' to find out how to do this.

The SET PRINTER command requires that you have installed the specified printer driver when you installed Epi Info. If you did not install this, you should run the install program again (you only need to install the printer section).

Check the status of your printer

You may find that nothing seems to happen after you have told ANALYSIS to print something. If so, follow this procedure:

1 Check that your printer is 'on-line'. If it is not, switch your printer 'on-line'.
2 If this is successful, then print again.
3 If this still does not work, check that data are being received by your printer. Many printers have a light which flashes to indicate that data are present.
4 Check whether there is a printer error (e.g. the printer may have run out of paper or be 'off-line'), correct if necessary and press 'resume' to carry on printing.

If all seems to be well, but a printout is still not forthcoming, type NEWPAGE at the EPI6> prompt and press ⟨ENTER⟩. This should flush out any unprinted pages.

Check the page size

The SET PAGE command controls the size of the page, which is measured in the number of characters wide, and the number of lines high. Normal settings are 23,80 for the screen and 66,80 for the printer.

If you wish to alter the normal settings, type:

Set page = ⟨number of characters wide⟩, ⟨number of lines high⟩ (e.g. SET PAGE = 72,88)

Getting the right values for your printer can be a matter of trial and error. It may be necessary to consult the full Epi Info manual and your printer manual if you cannot resolve difficulties using the steps described here.

Saving analysis output as a text file

If all else fails, you can save your output as a text file, which can be pasted into another program such as Microsoft Word, and then printed or incorporated into a Word document. This only works with text-based outputs, such as tables and listings – graphs and charts *cannot* be saved as a text file. If, for example, you want to save a frequency table of weight as a text file, type the following at the ANALYSIS command prompt:

1 ROUTE WEIGHT.TXT (instead of WEIGHT, you can use any word of up to eight characters, followed by .TXT)
2 Press ⟨ENTER⟩
3 FREQ WEIGHT
4 Press ⟨ENTER⟩
5 ROUTE SCREEN (this routes any *further* analysis to your screen, rather than it being added to the text file)
6 Press ⟨ENTER⟩

The file 'WEIGHT.TXT' will be saved in your EPI6 directory. To open it in Microsoft Word, do the following:

1 Click on 'Insert'.
2 Click on 'File'.
3 In the 'Look in' box, click on **C:** then **EPI6**.
4 In the 'Files of type' box, scroll down, and find 'Text files (*.txt)' – your file will be shown above.
5 Click on 'WEIGHT.TXT'.
6 Click on 'Insert' (press OK for a file conversion, *if prompted*).
7 The text file will now be inserted.

As mentioned previously, graphs produced within Epi Info cannot be directly transferred to a Word document. If you need to incorporate graphs from Epi Info data into a Word document, it is probably best to note the frequencies concerned, and use the 'chart' facility within Word to produce them. Although this sounds complicated and drawn out, it takes very little time in practice, and allows a great deal of flexibility in choosing the type of graph, as well as labelling and appearance.

Exporting and importing files

Exporting Epi Info files

1 Open the EXPORT program.
2 Type the input filename (this is the name of the existing Epi Info file you want to export e.g. DIABETES.REC) and press ⟨ENTER⟩.

3 Select the output format that you want to export the file as (e.g. LOTUS 1-2-3, dBASE 4, etc.). When you click on the format you want, a bold dot will appear at its side.
4 The output filename will be displayed in the 'Output filename' box, followed by the appropriate extension (e.g. DIABETES.WKS). You can change this filename if you wish.
5 Click on OK.
6 A box will appear on the screen, indicating that the export has taken place.
7 Click on OK.
8 The exported file will be placed in the EPI6 directory.
9 Click on CANCEL to return to the Epi Info main menu.

Opening exported data files in Microsoft Excel 2000

1 Open Microsoft Excel 2000.
2 Click on 'File'.
3 Click on 'Open'.
4 Select either 'Lotus 1-2-3 files' (recommended) or 'dBase files' in the 'Files of type' box.
5 Use the 'Look in' box to locate the file you wish to open (it will probably be in the EPI6 directory) and ensure its filename is displayed in the 'File name' box.
6 Click on 'Open'.

Saving Microsoft Excel 2000 files for import into Epi Info

1 Open the file in Microsoft Excel 2000.
2 Click on 'File'.
3 Click on 'Save as'.
4 Select a file format in the 'Save as type' box (e.g. WKS/WK1/WK3/ WK4 for Lotus 1-2-3, or DBF2/3/4 for dBase) – Lotus 1-2-3 format is recommended.
5 Use the 'Save in' box to select a directory to save the file in.
6 Click on 'Save'.

You may be alerted to the fact that the file you are saving may not retain certain features – you may wish to click on YES to leave it as it is. When closing the file in Excel, click NO to prevent saving the file in Excel format.

Importing Lotus 1-2-3 or dBASE files into Epi Info

1 Open the IMPORT program.
2 Select either LOTUS or dBASE from the options available.
3 Type the input filename (this is the name of the file you want to import into Epi Info, e.g. `A:DIABETES.WKS` or `C:\EPI6\WAITING.DBF`).
4 Type the output filename (this is the name of the Epi Info file you want to import the LOTUS or dBASE file into. This does not have to be an existing file – just type a suitable Epi Info name, e.g. `TEST.REC`) and press ⟨ENTER⟩.
5 Click on OK. The import will now take place.
6 Open the ANALYSIS program.
7 Type `READ` then press ⟨ENTER⟩.
8 Select the required file, and analyse the data as normal.
9 Click on CANCEL to return to the Epi Info main menu.

ANALYSIS can work directly with dBASE files. You may not need to use the IMPORT program to create a .REC file if you have data in dBASE format. If you want to import a file from Microsoft Excel or another program, first save the file as either a LOTUS 1-2-3 or dBASE format from within that program.

7

Basic statistics in Epi Info

When you use the TABLES or FREQ commands a variety of statistical information is displayed. This book cannot provide an in-depth guide to statistics, but if you would like to know more about this subject, some useful books on statistics are included within the bibliography.

Defining statistics

Statistics are used to describe and summarise information. Statistics has been defined as follows:

The science of assembling and interpreting numerical data.
(Bland, 1996)

The discipline concerned with the treatment of numerical data derived from groups of individuals.
(Armitage and Berry, 2002)

Some statistics simply describe data, and are called *descriptive statistics*. As well as just describing data, however, statistics can be used to actually draw *conclusions* or make *predictions* about what may happen in other subjects – these are called *inferential statistics*.

> 1 Antibiotics reduce the duration of viral throat infections by 1–2 days.
> 2 5% of women aged 30–49 consult their GP each year with heavy menstrual bleeding.
> 3 At our health centre, 50 patients were diagnosed with angina last year.
> Source: Stewart, 2002, p. 1

Examples 1 and 2 are inferential; though *all* may also be regarded as descriptive.

There are many ways of describing the data produced in an audit, and a brief explanation of some of the types of statistic produced by ANALYSIS appears below. Following this, we will see how Epi Info can be used for both descriptive and inferential statistics. Although explanations are included of how the statistics are calculated, Epi Info calculates all of the following statistics for you.

Types of data

There are two basic types of data:

- **Continuous**: each value can have a smaller value in between (e.g. height of 1.35 m) – **the value is being measured**.
- **Categorical**: each value is clearly separate from the next, with no fraction in between (e.g. number of children in a family, number of operations carried out), and can only have categories or whole numbers – **the value is being counted**.

Statistics shown in Epi Info tables

Data for some of the tables shown have been taken from the PATSAT file used in the patient satisfaction audit in Chapter 8. A frequency table for AGE is shown on p. 92.

Total

This adds up the number of records containing a value for the field being analysed. In the example table, the number of cases shown in the 'Total' column is **141**. This indicates that the ages of 141 separate patients have been recorded.

Sum

Adds up all of the values in the field being analysed. In the example, all of the ages recorded have been added up, and displayed under 'Sum'. This is shown in the 'Sum' column under the frequency table. The sum of all the ages in the example table is **4632**.

Maximum

The largest value in a field. The maximum age in the example table is **69**. This indicates that the maximum (or highest) age recorded is 69.

Minimum

The smallest value in a field. The minimum in the example table is **15**. This indicates that the minimum (or lowest) age recorded is 15.

Mean

This is another word for 'average'. Means are calculated by adding up all the values, and dividing by the number of items. They are useful for showing the *central tendency* of a group of numbers. The mean age for the example table is **32.851**. This indicates that the average of the recorded ages is 32.851 years. It has been calculated by taking the sum of all ages recorded (4632) and dividing it by the total number of ages recorded (141).

Note that the mean can be misleading if there are extreme values in the group. For example the mean of the group 1, 2, 3, 2, 4, 5, 19 is 5.143. Since only *one* of the values in the group is actually 5.143 or greater, the mean is not representative of the group. In this case, the median may be a better way of representing the data.

```
AGE   |   Freq    Percent      Cum.
------+-----------------------------
  15  |     3      2.1%        2.1%      ← minimum
  16  |     1      0.7%        2.8%
  17  |     3      2.1%        5.0%
  19  |     1      0.7%        5.7%
  21  |     6      4.3%        9.9%
  22  |     6      4.3%       14.2%
  23  |    11      7.8%       22.0%      ← mode
  24  |     5      3.5%       25.5%
  25  |     7      5.0%       30.5%
  26  |     7      5.0%       35.5%
  27  |     8      5.7%       41.1%
  28  |     5      3.5%       44.7%
  29  |     3      2.1%       46.8%
  30  |     5      3.5%       50.4%      ← median
  31  |     3      2.1%       52.5%
  32  |     7      5.0%       57.4%
  33  |     5      3.5%       61.0%      ← mean
  34  |     1      0.7%       61.7%        (32.851)
  35  |     3      2.1%       63.8%
  36  |     5      3.5%       67.4%
  37  |     5      3.5%       70.9%
  38  |     4      2.8%       73.8%
  39  |     5      3.5%       77.3%
  40  |     8      5.7%       83.0%
  44  |     1      0.7%       83.7%
  46  |     2      1.4%       85.1%
  47  |     2      1.4%       86.5%
  48  |     1      0.7%       87.2%
  49  |     3      2.1%       89.4%
  51  |     2      1.4%       90.8%
  52  |     1      0.7%       91.5%
  53  |     2      1.4%       92.9%
  54  |     1      0.7%       93.6%
  55  |     1      0.7%       94.3%
  56  |     2      1.4%       95.7%
  57  |     2      1.4%       97.2%
  58  |     1      0.7%       97.9%
  60  |     2      1.4%       99.3%
  69  |     1      0.7%      100.0%      ← maximum
------+-----------------------------
Total       141    100.0%              ← total
```

Total	Sum	Mean	Variance	Std Dev	Std Err
141	4632	32.851	125.785	11.215	0.945

Minimum	25%ile	Median	75%ile	Maximum	Mode
15.000	24.000	30.000	39.000	69.000	23.000

Median

This is the central value of a group of numbers which cuts off the bottom half of all the numbers. It is calculated by arranging all of the recorded numbers in order of magnitude, then taking the middle number.

If we arrange the numbers 1, 2, 3, 2, 4, 5 and 19 into numerical order, we get:

1, 2, 2, **3**, 4, 5, 19

The median is **3**, which is much more representative of the group than the mean (5.143). The median is not affected by extreme values and is usually typical of the data used.

If there is an even number of values, use the mean of the two central values:

19, 24, 26, 30, 31, 34

The median is $(26 + 30)/2 = \textbf{28}$. The median age in the example table is **30**.

Mode

This is the most frequently occurring value in a group of numbers or categories. In the example table the age 23 has been recorded more often than any of the other ages (11 times in all).

The mode is easy to find, requiring no mathematical calculation, and is usually typical of the data used. Because the mode only records the one most popular value, the others are not taken into account so it is not affected by extreme values.

The mode is most useful when 'categories' are being counted instead of numbers. For example, if you wanted to know the most frequently used health promotion clinic (e.g. 'smoking cessation', 'weight loss', 'healthy woman', 'healthy man', etc.) at your surgery, you would count up the attendances at all of them over a period, and find the one with the highest attendance. If there are two modes in a group of numbers, the group is said to be *bi-modal*. Note that Epi Info only displays the first mode in a multi-modal distribution, so it is always important to inspect the table as well as the 'mode' column.

25%ile and 75%ile

These are the 25th and 75th percentiles of a group of numbers. The 25th percentile is the point which cuts off the bottom quarter of the numbers in a group, in the same way as the median cuts off the bottom half (you could, in fact, say that the median is the 50th percentile). The 75th percentile is the point which cuts off the *top* quarter of the numbers.

For example, in the following set of numbers:

4, 5, **6**, 7, 7, **8**, 9, 9, **10**, 12, 14

the 25%ile is 6, the median is 8 and the 75%ile is 10.

In the Epi Info frequency table for ages (statistics summarised below), the '25%ile' and '75%ile' columns show their values to be 24 and 39 respectively.

Total	Sum	Mean	Variance	Std Dev	Std Err
141	4632	32.851	125.785	11.215	0.945
Minimum	**25%ile**	Median	**75%ile**	Maximum	Mode
15.000	**24.000**	30.000	**39. 000**	69.000	23.000

Standard deviation

This is used to find out how much a group of numbers differ from their mean. The larger the standard deviation, the more the numbers differ from their mean.

For example, one small group of patients in a particular outpatients clinic may wait for a mean time of 11 minutes to be seen by a doctor, and the standard deviation from the mean for this group is 5.701. Individual waiting times vary widely – from 7 minutes up to 21 minutes. There is wide variation between these waiting times, and they are quite widely spread out from their mean. These waiting times are therefore *heterogeneous* or dissimilar.

Another group of patients from the same clinic on another day may also have a mean waiting time of 11 minutes, but their standard deviation is 0.707. This is much less than the first group's standard deviation of 5.701. Looking at this group's actual waiting times, it can be seen that they only vary from 10 to 12 minutes. Waiting times for the second group are more *homogeneous* – meaning that the data are more similar to each other. They are less widely spread out around their mean than the first group.

Let's look at the actual waiting times recorded for each group:

Group	Time 1	Time 2	Time 3	Time 4	Time 5	Mean	Standard deviation
1	10	7	8	9	21	11	5.701
2	11	11	10	11	12	11	0.707

The above figures are shown in the following Epi Info frequency distributions:

```
Group 1

TIME  | Freq  Percent   Cum.
------+-----------------------
  7   |   1    20.0%    20.0%
  8   |   1    20.0%    40.0%
  9   |   1    20.0%    60.0%
 10   |   1    20.0%    80.0%
 21   |   1    20.0%   100.0%
------+-----------------------
Total |   5   100.0%


       Total         Sum       Mean   Variance    Std Dev    Std Err
         5            55     11.000     32.500      5.701      2.550

     Minimum       25%ile     Median    75%ile    Maximum       Mode
      7.000        8.000      9.000     10.000     21.000      7.000



Group 2

TIME  | Freq  Percent   Cum.
------+-----------------------
 10   |   1    20.0%    20.0%
 11   |   3    60.0%    80.0%
 12   |   1    20.0%   100.0%
------+-----------------------
Total |   5   100.0%


       Total         Sum       Mean   Variance    Std Dev    Std Err
         5            55     11.000      0.500      0.707      0.316

     Minimum       25%ile     Median    75%ile    Maximum       Mode
     10.000       11.000     11.000     11.000     12.000     11.000
```

You can see that the data in Group 1 are much more spread out than the data in Group 2. This difference in standard deviations can be explained by the fact that although most patients in Group 1 waited a very short time, one patient had to wait for a long time – 21 minutes.

Although this one 'outlier' waiting time is not representative of the whole group, it has a big effect on the overall results, and strongly affects the mean and standard deviation. Several patients from Group 2 actually waited longer than Group 1 patients, though the difference between the waiting times in Group 2 is very slight.

In the frequency table for ages, the standard deviation of the ages recorded is 11.215. This suggests that the minimum and maximum ages differ quite substantially from the mean age (or that there is a broad range of ages), which is confirmed by the summary statistics:

Total	Sum	Mean	Variance	Std Dev	Std Err
141	4632	32.851	125.785	11.215	0.945
Minimum	**25%ile**	Median	**75%ile**	**Maximum**	Mode
15.000	**24.000**	30.000	**39.000**	**69.000**	23.000

Variance

This is worked out in the last stage of the standard deviation calculation. The square root of the variance produces the standard deviation.

In the example above, the square root of the variance (125.785) equals 11.215 (use a calculator to work it out – your answer will probably be 11.215391, or 11.215 to 3 decimal places).

The variance on its own will not be useful for any of the topics covered by this book. It is, however, used in some other functions of Epi Info, which require you to enter in the variance (for example, there are functions in the EPITABLE program that allow you to directly compare means or variances).

Standard error

Standard error is another term for the standard deviation of a *sampling distribution* (this means a frequency distribution of samples), rather than just a sample. If, for example, we took a large number of samples of a particular size from a population and recorded the mean for each sample, we could calculate the standard deviation of all their means – called the *standard error* (or sometimes SE). Because it is based on a very large number of (theoretical) samples, it should be more precise and therefore smaller than the standard deviation. Standard error is used in a range of statistical calculations, but a standard error value on its own (e.g. 0.945 in the above example) is of little use to you, as Epi Info calculates most things automatically.

If you are interested, the standard error can be calculated by dividing the standard deviation by the square root of the sample size. In the above table, the square root of the sample size ('total' = 141) is 11.87 – the standard deviation (11.215) divided by 11.87 is 0.945 (to 3 decimal places).

Inferential statistics in Epi Info

As discussed earlier, inferential statistics allow us to draw *conclusions* or make *predictions* about what may happen in other subjects. To do this, we need to consider the issues of *sampling* and *hypotheses*.

Sampling

It is important to understand the difference between populations and samples. A **population** can be defined as *every subject* in a country, a town, a district or other group being studied. Imagine you are carrying out an audit of postoperative infection rates in a hospital during the past year. The population for your study (called the **target population**) is *everyone* in that hospital who had surgery in that year. Using this population, a **sampling frame** can be constructed. This is a list of every person in the population from whom your sample will be taken. Each individual in the sampling frame is usually assigned a number, which can be used in the actual sampling process.

If thousands of operations have been carried out during the year, there may not be time to look at every case history. It may therefore only be possible to look at a smaller group (e.g. 200) of these patients. This smaller group is a **sample**.

A **statistic** is a value calculated from a **sample**, which describes a particular feature. It is only ever an **estimate** of the true value. For example, if we take a sample of 100 patients who had surgery during 2001, we might find that seven developed a postoperative infection. A different sample of 100 patients, however, might identify 11 postoperative infections, and another may find eight infections. We will almost always find such differences between samples, and these are called **sampling variations**.

A scientific study usually aims to be able to generalise the results to the population as a whole. So we need a sample that is **representative** of the population. While audits are not always carried out with this aim in mind, a representative sample will make the results more accurate and credible. Going back to our example of postoperative infections, it is rarely possible to collect data on *everyone* in a population. Methods therefore exist to collect enough data to be reasonably sure that results will be accurate and applicable to the whole population. The random sampling methods in the next section are among those used to achieve this.

So we often have to rely on a sample for an audit, because it may be impractical to collect data from *everyone* in the population. A sample can be used to *estimate* quantities in the population as a whole, and to calculate the likely accuracy of the estimate. This is important, since increasing the sample size will tend to increase the accuracy of your estimate, while a smaller sample size will usually decrease the accuracy. Furthermore, the right sample size is vital to allow you to detect a statistically significant effect, if one exists. The calculation of sample size and some sampling techniques for clinical audit are discussed in Chapter 8.

Many sampling techniques exist, and these can be divided into **non-random** and **random**. These are discussed further in Chapter 8.

Probability

Scale of probability:

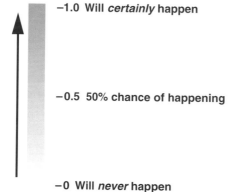

–1.0 Will *certainly* happen

–0.5 50% chance of happening

–0 Will *never* happen

- For example, when tossing a coin, there is a 50% chance of getting a head

- Probabilities are usually expressed in **decimal** format – 50% becomes 0.5, 10% is 0.1 and 5% is 0.05

- The probability of getting a head when tossing the coin is therefore 0.5

- A probability can *never* be more than 1.0, or negative

Confidence intervals

Medical literature often mentions '95% confidence intervals'. This means the range within which the true size of an effect (never exactly known) lies with a given degree of certainty. This is the interval which, with 95% probability, is likely to contain the true value in the population. They are usually written as: 95% CI 75 (70 → 84).

For example, if you want to examine the effect of a new antihypertensive drug in your clinic, you might treat a random sample of half your hypertensive patients with the new drug, and the other half with a standard treatment. The results might show that the mean systolic blood pressure (BP) of patients on the new treatment is 75 mmHg, compared with a mean of 88 mmHg for the other patients.

The problem is that we are dealing with a sample of patients, and do not know what the result might have been if we had been able to measure the systolic BP of *every* hypertensive patient in the whole population. The confidence interval estimates, with 95% confidence, the range where the systolic BP of the population might *really* be in the population.

In the example above, the 95% CI is 75 (70 → 84). Even at the highest end of the range, the estimated mean BP of 84 is still lower than the mean of 88 in the group of patients receiving standard treatment. This indicates that the new treatment is *significantly* better than the standard treatment. If the 95% CI had been 75 (67 → 91), this would show that at the highest end of the range, the estimate is *worse* than the standard treatment; in this case, although the mean of the new treatment looks better than the standard treatment, it could actually be less effective than the standard treatment.

Hypotheses

A **hypothesis** is an *unproved theory*, made as a starting point for an investigation – for example 'patients who take drug A will have better outcomes than those who take drug B' or 'drug A is better than drug B'. The hypothesis that 'drug A is better than drug B' is often written as H_1.

For every hypothesis there is a **null hypothesis**. In the above scenarios, the null hypothesis is that 'the outcomes of patients taking drug A will be *no different* to those who take drug B' or that 'drug A is *no better* than drug B'. Scientific experiments tend to adopt a somewhat sceptical attitude and normally use the null hypothesis to try and disprove the real hypothesis. The null hypothesis is often written as H_0.

If drug A proves significantly better than drug B, the null hypothesis (H_0) is rejected, and the **alternative hypothesis** (H_1) is accepted.

The problem is, how do we know how much better the difference or size of effect needs to be to reach statistical significance? In practice, we assess the probability that the effect we found (or a more extreme effect) would have occurred if the null hypothesis were true. If the probability is low, it follows that the effect may be due to the effectiveness of the treatment – or possibly some other cause. To make this assessment, we need to calculate a **test statistic**, and use this to determine the probability (expressed as a **p value**). If the p value is **0.05 or less**, this is usually considered to be statistically significant. This process is often called **hypothesis testing**.

In this section, we will carry out three different hypothesis tests:

- the paired *t*-test
- the independent *t*-test
- the chi-squared test.

The paired t-test

This test is used for the difference between the means of two paired measurements. In this case, data are naturally paired or matched, such as weight measurements from the *same subjects* at a six-month interval or data relative to twins or couples.

For example, a GP wants to assess how effective a new drug is at reducing diastolic blood pressure in 12 of her hypertensive patients. The dataset below shows diastolic blood pressure before and after these patients received the new drug:

```
Patient       |       Old       |       New
------------+------------------+-----------------
1           |       96        |       87
2           |       90        |       75
3           |       95        |       85
4           |       105       |       80
5           |       100       |       75
6           |       105       |       85
7           |       95        |       75
8           |       110       |       85
9           |       100       |       80
10          |       115       |       85
11          |       95        |       75
12          |       105       |       80
```

You can see that patients all have lower diastolic blood pressure after receiving the new drug. Our null hypothesis is that there is *no* statistically significant difference between the mean blood pressure of those taking the new drug compared with the mean blood pressure on their previous treatments. The alternative hypothesis is that there *is* a statistically significant difference. We are comparing the mean diastolic blood pressure *before* receiving the new drug to the mean *after* receiving it.

Let's carry out this test as follows:

1 Start Epi Info
2 In EPED, type the following:
    PATIENT # #
    OLD # # #
    NEW # # #
3 Press **F9**, and save it as BLOOD.QES
4 Press **F10** to exit from EPED
5 Go into ENTER
6 Type BLOOD and press ⟨ENTER⟩
7 Select option 2, then type BLOOD again
8 Press ⟨ENTER⟩ twice
9 Type in the data from the dataset above
10 Press **F10** to exit from ENTER
11 Go into ANALYSIS
12 Type READ BLOOD and press ⟨ENTER⟩
13 Type DEFINE DIFFER # # # and press ⟨ENTER⟩

14 Type DIFFER = OLD – NEW and press ⟨ENTER⟩

15 Type FREQ DIFFER/N and press ⟨ENTER⟩ (*typing* /N *after* DIFF *displays only the statistics, omitting the individual values*).

The output on your screen should look like this:

```
DIFFER

        Total        Sum       Mean    Variance     Std Dev     Std Err
          12          244     20.333      40.424       6.358       1.835

      Minimum      25%ile     Median      75%ile     Maximum        Mode
        9.000      17.500     20.000      25.000      30.000      20.000

Student's "t", testing whether mean differs from zero.
T statistic = 11.078,   df =    11   p-value = 0.00000
```

The p value is *less than* 0.05, so there is a *significant difference* between the diastolic blood pressures. In this case, the difference is quite extreme, and the p value is very small indeed (less than 0.00001). If you were reporting this, you could write:

There was a significant difference between the diastolic blood pressures of the patients taking the new drug and previous treatments (t = 11.078, p < 0.00001).

The independent t-test

This is used where data are collected from groups that are unrelated, such as the length at age one year of a group of infants who were breast-fed, compared with a group who were not breast-fed. The test compares the means of the two independent samples.

As part of a diabetes audit at a district hospital, a diabetologist is interested to ascertain whether there is any difference in diabetic control (measured using HbA1c levels) between female patients and male patients. The values of ten male and ten female patients are recorded. The dataset is shown below:

Group 1 (Males)	Group 2 (Females)
8.6	7.9
5.4	4.9
10.7	7.6
5.5	10.8
4.5	6.1
6.9	9.9
5.8	7.2
5.1	5.6
4.4	7.3
11.1	10.3

1 Start Epi Info
2 In EPED, type the following:
   LEVEL # #.#
   GROUP #
3 Press **F9**, and save it as CONTROL.QES
4 Press **F10** to exit from EPED
5 Go into ENTER
6 Type CONTROL and press ⟨ENTER⟩
7 Select option 2, and press ⟨ENTER⟩
8 Type CONTROL again
9 Press ⟨ENTER⟩ twice
10 Type in the data from the dataset above – enter each HbA1c level in the 'level' field, and the corresponding group number in the 'group' field
11 Press **F10** to exit from ENTER
12 Go into ANALYSIS
13 Type READ CONTROL and press ⟨ENTER⟩
14 Type MEANS LEVEL GROUP and press ⟨ENTER⟩

The output on your screen should look like this (the top half of the output has been omitted):

```
GROUP           Obs       Total       Mean     Variance    Std Dev
1                10         68        6.800      6.171       2.484
2                10         78        7.760      4.049       2.012
Difference                            -0.960

GROUP         Minimum     25%ile      Median    75%ile     Maximum        Mode
1               4.400      5.100       5.650     8.600      11.100        4.400
2               4.900      6.100       7.450     9.900      10.800        4.900

                                  ANOVA
                    (For normally distributed data only)

Variation       SS    df         MS    F statistic    p-value     t-value
Between        4.608   1        4.608      0.902      0.354897    0.949590
Within        91.984  18        5.110
Total         96.592  19

                 Bartlett's test for homogeneity of variance
        Bartlett's chi square =   0.376  deg freedom = 1   p-value = 0.539955

            The variances are homogeneous with 95% confidence.
    If samples are also normally distributed, ANOVA results can be used.

Mann-Whitney or Wilcoxon Two-Sample Test (Kruskal-Wallis test for two groups)

Kruskal-Wallis H (equivalent to Chi square) =       1.463
                       Degrees of freedom =            1
                                 p value =        0.226476
```

The text beneath the ANOVA results indicates that these results can be used. You can see that the p value is therefore **0.354897**.

The p value is *more than* 0.05, so there is *no* significant difference between HbA1c values in males and females. If you were reporting this, you could write:

The difference between the mean HbA1c levels of men compared to women was not significant (t = 0.949590, p = 0.354897).

The chi-squared test

We have so far looked at hypothesis tests for continuous data (data for variables that have continuous values, such as height, weight or blood pressure), from which summary statistics such as means and medians can be calculated. When we have only categorical data (data for variables that are not continuous, but are arranged into categories such as ethnic group, gender or yes/no answers), however, means and medians cannot be produced. For example, you cannot calculate the mean of a group of colours.

The chi-squared test (chi is pronounced 'ki', as in 'kind', and is normally written as χ^2) overcomes this problem, allowing hypothesis testing for categorical data. Instead of testing for a difference between means, it tests whether there is a significant **association** between two categorical variables.

For example, an epidemiological study examined several possible causes for an outbreak of food poisoning at a large party. Everyone who attended was asked a series of questions, including whether they were ill, and what types of food they ate while at the party. In this exercise, we will focus on whether they were ill, and explore what food was responsible for the disease outbreak. We will use a ready-made dataset, which is included with Epi Info.

1 Start Epi Info
2 Go into ANALYSIS
3 Type READ OSWEGO and press ⟨ENTER⟩

Let's start by seeing whether there is any association between eating spinach and being ill:

• Type TABLES SPINACH ILL and press ⟨ENTER⟩

The output on the screen should look like this:

```
ILL
SPINACH     |      +      -  | Total
------------+----------------+------
         +  |     26     17  |    43
         -  |     20     12  |    32
------------+----------------+------
     Total  |     46     29  |    75


                        Single Table Analysis

Odds ratio
0.92
Cornfield 95% confidence limits for OR                  0.32 < OR <   2.63
Maximum likelihood estimate of OR (MLE)
0.92
Exact 95% confidence limits for MLE                     0.32 < OR <   2.59
Exact 95% Mid-P limits for MLE                          0.35 < OR <   2.38
Probability of MLE <=  0.92 if population OR = 1.0       0.52525029

RISK RATIO(RR)(Outcome:ILL=+; Exposure:SPINACH=+)  0.97
95% confidence limits for RR                            0.67 < RR <   1.39
              Ignore risk ratio if case control study

                         Chi-Squares   P-values
                         -----------   --------

           Uncorrected:       0.03     0.85795437
       Mantel-Haenszel:       0.03     0.85889451
       Yates corrected:       0.00     0.95157827
```

The 2×2 table at the start of the output shows frequencies for exposure (spinach) displayed down the left-hand side, and the outcome (illness) across the top. Ignore the output in the middle, and concentrate on the bottom section, headed chi-squares and p values. The *uncorrected chi-squared value* is 0.03, and the p value is 0.8580.

The p value is *more than* 0.05, so there is *no significant association* between eating spinach and being ill.

You can explore other exposures by typing TABLES followed by a different exposure (e.g. SALAD) and ILL. In this case: TABLES MILK ILL or TABLES CAKES ILL, for example. Finally, try vanilla (ice cream) – type TABLES VANILLA ILL.

```
                            ILL
VANILLA         |      +      -  |  Total
----------------+----------------+------
            +   |     43     11  |    54
            -   |      3     18  |    21
----------------+----------------+------
     Total      |     46     29  |    75

                     Single Table Analysis

Odds ratio
23.45
Cornfield 95% confidence limits for OR              5.07 < OR < 125.19*
                                                  *May be inaccurate
Maximum likelihood estimate of OR (MLE)
22.15
Exact 95% confidence limits for MLE                5.22 < OR < 138.39
Exact 95% Mid-P limits for MLE                      5.93 < OR < 109.15
Probability of MLE >= 22.15 if population OR = 1.0      0.00000026

RISK RATIO(RR)(Outcome:ILL=+; Exposure:VANILLA=+)            5.57
95% confidence limits for RR                     1.94 < RR <   16.03

              Ignore risk ratio if case control study

                        Chi-Squares    P-values
                        -----------    --------

          Uncorrected:      27.22      0.00000018 <---
          Mantel-Haenszel:  26.86      0.00000022 <---
          Yates corrected:  24.54      0.00000073 <---
```

This time, the uncorrected chi-squared value is 27.22, with a p value of 0.00000018. The p value can also be written as $p < 0.0001$. You can see that in this test, Epi Info has marked all of the significant p values with an arrow (<---). As the p value is less than 0.05, there is a significant association between eating vanilla (ice cream) and being ill. If you were reporting this, you could write:

There was a significant association between eating ice cream and being ill ($\chi^2 = 27.22$, $p < 0.0001$).

The Yates' corrected chi-squared value is 24.54 – Yates' correction gives a more conservative estimate, and is useful when small samples are used. You can see that the p value is larger, but in this case is still significant. It therefore appears that the ice cream caused this outbreak of food poisoning.

Chi-squared is more accurate when large frequencies are used. If the frequencies are too small, the chi-squared test may not be valid, and therefore cannot be used. The screen output will indicate this, where necessary, displaying the following message: 'AN EXPECTED VALUE IS

<5. CHI SQUARE IS NOT VALID'. **When this happens, the results shown cannot be used, even if they appear to be significant.**

Under some circumstances (when variables which each have only *two* possible answers are used, e.g. male/female and yes/no), Epi Info may be able to calculate **Fisher's exact test**. Where applicable, the following message is displayed: 'AN EXPECTED VALUE IS LESS THAN 5, RECOMMEND FISHER EXACT RESULTS', and these results will be shown. The Fisher's exact test gives a p value which is interpreted in the same way as usual.

When there are variables with *more* than two possible answers, it may be possible to regroup the data to create fewer columns. Doing this will increase the cell frequencies, which may then be large enough to meet the requirements of the test. For example, if you have four age groups (0–7, 8–14, 15–21, 22–28), it might be reasonable to combine these to produce two age groups (0–14 and 15–28). Regrouping data into fewer categories is a compromise, however, as the precision allowed by having so many categories will be reduced.

8

Using Epi Info for sampling and calculating sample sizes

Random and non-random sampling

We have already discussed populations and samples, *see* p. 97. Many sampling techniques exist, and these can be divided into **non-random** and **random**. In random sampling (also called **probability sampling**), everyone in the sampling frame has an equal probability of being chosen. This aims to make the sample more representative of the population from which it is drawn. There are several methods of random sampling, and some of these are discussed later in this section. Non-random sampling (also called **non-probability sampling**) does not have these aims, but is usually easier and more convenient to carry out.

Non-random sampling

Convenience or **opportunistic sampling** is the crudest kind of non-random sampling. This involves selecting the most convenient group available (e.g. using the first ten patients you see during morning surgery). It is simple to carry out, but is unlikely to result in a sample that is either representative of the population or replicable.

A commonly used **non-random** method of sampling is **quota sampling**. This is where a pre-defined number (or quota) of people who meet certain criteria are surveyed. For example, an interviewer may be tasked with interviewing 25 people in an outpatient waiting area on a weekday morning – the instructions may specify that seven of these should be aged under 30, ten should be aged between 30 and 45, and eight should be aged over 45. While this is a convenient sampling method, it will not necessarily produce results that are representative of all people who attend outpatients.

Random sampling

Random selection of the sample is another important issue. In random sampling everyone in the sampling frame has an equal probability of being chosen. For a sample to be truly representative of the population, a random sample should be taken. Random sampling can also help to minimise **bias**. Bias can be defined as an effect that produces results which are *systematically* different from the *true* values.

For example, imagine you are carrying out an audit on angina management. You have 300 patients with angina and want to find out what proportion have been given advice on smoking cessation. You might make a list of all these patients and decide to examine the records of the first 50 on the list. If most are found to have received smoking cessation advice, are the *other* 250 likely to be similar? Furthermore, what if someone accuses you of 'fixing' the sample, by only picking patients who you *know* have received this advice? If you use a random sampling system, such doubts can be avoided.

There are many different random sampling systems, but one simple method is to use a **random number list**. Epi Info can generate a random number list, and instructions on how to do this are shown below. For example, if you want a random sample of 50 from a population of 300, you could list all 300 subjects and assign a number to each. Then use the numbers on the random number list which match the numbers you have assigned. This produces a **simple random sample**.

Producing a random number list using Epi Info

To produce a random number list in Epi Info, follow these instructions:

- From the Epi Info main menu, open the EPITABLE CALCULATOR.
- Click on the SAMPLE menu, on the menu bar along the top of the window.
- Click on RANDOM NUMBER LIST.

- Type in *how many* random numbers you need (e.g. 50) and press ⟨ENTER⟩.
- Choose the *minimum* range of numbers you require (usually one) and press ⟨ENTER⟩.
- Select the *maximum* range of numbers needed (e.g. 300) and press ⟨ENTER⟩.
- Click on CALCULATE – a window showing your random number list will appear.
- To print this list, click on FILES and then click on PRINT.
- Press ⟨ESC⟩ or click on the green square (in the top left-hand corner of the window) to exit – before exiting you have the option to save the list.

Using this method to generate 50 random numbers from 300 produces a list. An example is shown below:

8	12	14	22	24
27	33	37	49	55
67	78	79	93	95
98	104	108	113	116
125	128	129	133	138
143	158	163	167	169
171	173	176	184	193
203	212	218	219	221
224	225	230	232	249
264	272	273	283	285

Stratified sampling

It can be useful to employ **stratified sampling** to randomly select subjects from different strata or groups. Visualise an audit to examine whether patients with diabetes have received an eye check. Because Asian residents are more likely to get diabetes, it might be desirable to examine possible variations in healthcare between Asian and non-Asian patients. A simple random sample of patients on a list would almost certainly produce very few Asian patients, as most localities have a low proportion of Asian residents. In such a case, we could stratify our sample by dividing patients into Asian and non-Asian, and then take a random sample of each.

Systematic sampling

A less random, but nevertheless useful, approach is to use a **systematic sampling** scheme. In this method, a number is assigned to every record, and then every n^{th} record is selected from a list. For example, if you want to systematically select 50 of your 300 patients with angina:

1 Obtain a list of all 300 patients with angina (this is your sampling frame).
2 As $300/50 = 6$, you will be taking every sixth patient.
3 Choose a number randomly between 1 and 6 as a starting point.
4 Take every sixth patient thereafter; e.g. if your starting point is 4, you will take patients number 4, 10, 16, 22, 28, 34, etc.

By doing this, you are using the list rather than your own judgement to select the patients. Look at the list carefully before you start selecting. For example, choosing every tenth patient in a list of married couples may well result in every selected person being male or every person being female (Donaldson and Donaldson, 2000).

Sample size

In addition to using the correct method of sampling, there are also ways of calculating a sample size that is appropriate. As mentioned earlier, increasing the sample size will tend to increase the accuracy of your estimate, while a smaller sample size will usually decrease the accuracy. Also, the right sample size is vital to allow you to detect a statistically significant effect, if one exists. The appropriate sample size can be calculated using one of several formulae, according to the type of study and data being collected. Further elements of sample size calculation are discussed more fully in other books (*see* Bibliography). If statistical significance is not vital, a sample size of between 50 and 100 may suffice for many purposes.

Calculating sample size using Epi Info

When planning an audit project, it is important to collect data from as many subjects as possible to help ensure that your results will be accurate and representative. For example, if you are doing an audit on hypertension, you may feel it necessary to examine the records of all your hypertensive patients so the result will be representative of the whole group. If you look at only half of the group to see if their BP has been checked in the past 12 months and find that most have been recorded, how do you know that the other half have never had their BP taken? If you use only a small sample of patients, how can you be sure that only 'good' or 'bad' cases have been selected?

The problem is that looking at every record can be immensely time-consuming. If, however, you choose not to view each and every one you risk losing accuracy, thus making the whole project ineffective and invalid.

Providing your audit uses simple criterion-based questions (e.g. yes/no, present/absent, etc.), the following method will save you time, especially if the audit is large.

While audits do not usually restrict themselves to asking only yes/no questions, it is usually possible to identify one crucial area that an audit is evaluating which could prove the basis for the primary criterion. For example, a patient satisfaction audit may be asking several questions, but its primary aim is to determine whether or not patients are satisfied with the overall service. One primary criterion and standard should therefore be set which can be explicitly answered by just one yes/no or present/absent-type answer. Any other information collected will be useful, but is secondary to that one crucial question. If you can identify one such question, this method can safely be used for your audit.

The method presented here is suited to the collection of categorical data. This means that there are discrete categories of data, and each category is completely separate from the next. Examples are surnames, ethnic groups or genders.

Just follow these four steps:

1 Find out the total number in the group being studied.
2 Decide the confidence level you need.
3 Use Epi Info to calculate the sample size required.
4 Select the patients/records randomly.

Please note that this method is not suitable for continuous data, such as the range of body mass index (BMI) across a population. For situations like this, it is advisable to consult a statistician, or someone with advanced statistical skills.

Total number in group (population)

This relates to the number of patients who have the condition you are studying. If you are looking at diabetic patients, you will be wasting your time by looking at the records of every single patient registered with your hospital or practice, as you only want those who have been diagnosed with diabetes. If your register says you have 80 diabetic patients, then the total number in the group being studied is 80.

Confidence level

How confident do you need to be that the results are representative of the whole of your patient group? Scientists and statisticians tend to use confidence levels of 95% or higher, but levels of 90% may be sufficient for your needs. In any event, you need to make a compromise between absolute accuracy and the time available to collect all the data. For example:

- Using a 95% confidence level with the sample size shown, you can be 95% confident that results obtained will be representative.
- Using a 90% confidence level with the sample size shown, you can be 90% confident that results obtained will be representative.

The first option offers the higher percentage accuracy, but a larger sample size is required than for the second option, which gives a lower accuracy but requires a smaller sample size. Other higher or lower confidence levels (e.g. 85% or 99%) may also be used.

Sample size calculations with STATCALC

The sample size calculations used by STATCALC assume:

- The sample to be taken is a simple random (or otherwise representative) sample. A systematic sample, such as every other person on a clinic list, is acceptable only if the sample is representative.
- The question being asked must have a yes/no or other two-choice (also called dichotomous) answer leading to a proportion of the population (e.g. the number of 'yes' answers divided by the sample populations) as the final result.

Suppose you wish to investigate whether or not the true proportion of patients satisfied with a particular service is 80%. You plan to take a random or systematic sample of the population to estimate the prevalence. You would like 95% confidence that the true proportion (i.e. the proportion you would find if you surveyed the entire clinic population) will fall within the confidence interval calculated from your sample.
In STATCALC:

1 Select SAMPLE SIZE & POWER.
2 Select POPULATION SURVEY.
3 Enter the **size of population** (e.g. **15 000**).
4 Enter the **expected frequency** (an estimate of the true prevalence, e.g. **80%** – your minimum standard).
5 Enter the **worst acceptable result** (e.g. **75%**). This is one of the

confidence limits around the estimated sample proportion, indicating that the confidence interval you select will be accurate to within plus or minus 5% of your minimum standard. You therefore take five off your minimum standard percentage and use this number as the 'worst acceptable result'. The other confidence limit (85% in this case) is calculated automatically by the program. For increased accuracy, you may wish to use a confidence limit of plus or minus 2.5%, in which case you would enter 77.5% as your 'worst acceptable result'.

The program then calculates and displays sample sizes for several different confidence levels.

Sample size calculations are a rough guide based on assuming a specific value for the true population proportion, the variability in the sample estimate and its confidence limit. Many other factors, such as cost, number of subjects available, rates of non-response and the accuracy of data collection and entry, should also be considered.

More on selecting patients for the audit

Once you have determined the sample size required, it is important to be careful about selecting the actual records of individuals involved. For the audit to be truly representative, avoiding bias, these should be randomly distributed.

In the following example of a patient satisfaction audit (Example 1), questionnaires could be given to *every* patient attending the clinic, spread over several clinic sessions, until 137 completed questionnaires have been returned. This is 'random' because at the start of the audit you do not know who will be attending.

In the following example of an audit of hypertension (Example 2), you need to look at records for 85 of your 257 patients with hypertension. A good method is to obtain a list of all these patients and then use a random number list or a systematic sample, selecting every third record (257 divided by 85 = 3.02) to select your sample.

When you perform a re-audit on any subject, it is advisable to use exactly the same methods and criteria as before. So long as the conditions of the audit are the same you do not necessarily need to look at exactly the same patients again.

The method described here can save you a considerable amount of time in collecting data for an audit, while maintaining a good level of accuracy. Remember that such audits should rely on simple criterion-based questions.

Examples

Example 1: patient satisfaction audit

Aims

The St Elsewhere's GUM clinic sees around 15000 patients per year. This audit aims to improve the service at a genito-urinary medicine clinic. This will be done by assessing patient satisfaction with various aspects of the services provided and, by analysis of responses, considering whether any improvements should be made. The patient questionnaire will contain questions on several areas of activity, but the crucial question centres on patients' satisfaction with the overall service required.

Criteria and standards

At least 90% of patients should be satisfied or very satisfied with the following aspects of the service:

- reading material in waiting rooms
- information displayed in waiting rooms
- condition of the waiting rooms
- overall service received
- their welcome on arrival
- medical treatment received
- nursing treatment
- health advice received
- information about diagnosis.

At least 80% of patients should state that they would recommend the clinic to a friend.
   A 95% confidence level is required.

Methodology

For a period of one week, every patient attending the clinic will be asked to fill in a short questionnaire and return it to reception before leaving.

Data analysis and evaluation

The data will be entered using Epi Info and results produced. These will be compared with the standards originally set, and conclusions will be drawn as to whether any improvements should be made. A poster summarising the results of the audit and any changes made as a result of it will be displayed in the waiting room, for patients to see.

The audit will be repeated in 12 months, to re-evaluate patient satisfaction and assess whether any changes have been effective.

We will use Epi Info to calculate the sample size required for a population of 15 000.

From the PROGRAMS menu:

1 Select STATCALC
2 Select SAMPLE SIZE & POWER
3 Select POPULATION SURVEY
4 Type the size of population – 15000
5 Type 90 in EXPECTED FREQUENCY (your minimum standard for 'overall satisfaction')
6 Type 85 in WORST ACCEPTABLE RESULT (allowing for a possible 5% error for your minimum standard)
7 Press **F4**

A choice of six sample sizes will be displayed, depending on the confidence level required – 80%, 90%, 95%, 99%, 99.9% and 99.99%.

Read off the required sample size for 95% confidence (**137**). Data collection for this audit will therefore be complete when 137 questionnaire forms have been handed in. The sample can be regarded as being 'randomly' selected because *every* patient attending the clinic will be asked to participate, thus avoiding bias.

If you wish to find sample sizes required for different population sizes, use the arrow keys to move the cursor up to POPULATION SIZE, enter the new size and press ⟨ENTER⟩ to recalculate. You may find that Epi Info will not list the sample sizes until the size of population figure has been altered. If this happens, change the figure, perform the calculation, then change it back again to the figure you require and recalculate.

When you have calculated your sample size, press **F10** until you return to the Epi Info menu.

Example 2: audit of hypertension

Aims

This audit aims to ensure that all of the practice's 257 patients with hypertension are receiving a high quality of care.

Criteria and standards

- At least 95% of all the practice's patients with hypertension should have been reviewed within the last 12 months.
- A standard of at least 80% should be attained for each of the other areas being studied:
  - all patients should have had their blood pressure recorded within the past 12 months
  - all patients should have had their weight and height measured and recorded within the last 12 months
  - all patients should have had their smoking status and alcohol intake recorded within the last 12 months.

Methodology

All of the practice's patients with hypertension will be identified using the practice computer, and a random sample of their records will be examined to determine whether the appropriate checks have been recorded as being carried out. The specific sample size will be calculated using Epi Info's sample size calculation program (STATCALC). A confidence level of 99% is required.

Data analysis and evaluation

The data will be entered using Epi Info and results produced. These will be compared with the standards originally set and conclusions will be drawn as to whether any improvements should be made. The audit will be repeated in 12 months, to re-evaluate this area and assess whether any changes have been effective.

We will therefore use Epi Info to calculate the sample size required for a population of 257. From the PROGRAMS menu:

1 Select STATCALC
2 Select SAMPLE SIZE & POWER
3 Select POPULATION SURVEY
4 Type the size population – 257
5 Type 95 in EXPECTED FREQUENCY (your minimum standard for '12-month review')
6 Type 90 in WORST ACCEPTABLE RESULT (allowing for a possible 5% error for your minimum standard)
7 Press **F4**

A choice of six sample sizes will be displayed, depending on the confidence level required – 80%, 90%, 95%, 99%, 99.9% and 99.99%.

Read off the required sample size for 99% confidence (**85**). You therefore need to look at records for 85 of your 257 patients with hypertension.

When you have calculated your sample size, press **F10** until you return to the Epi Info menu.

9

Epi Info advanced tutorial

This tutorial concentrates on the more advanced facilities available in ANALYSIS. We will begin by creating a simple dataset. It could form the basis of a larger health promotion questionnaire, and you can add to or change the fields if you wish to use it for a real audit project. Each section has some questions, with answers at the end of this chapter.

Start EPED and type the following questionnaire:

```
Health Promotion Questionnaire
--------------------------------------------------------------

1. What is your date of birth {dob}? <dd/mm/yyyy>

2. What is your gender {sex}? (M or F) <A>

3. What is your {height}? (in metres) #.##

4. What is your {weight}? (in Kg) ###.#

5. What is your {occupation}? <AAAAAAAAAAAAAAAAAAAA>

--------------------------------------------------------------
```

Save the questionnaire (**F9**) as HEALTH.QES

Creating the data-entry system

Start ENTER and specify the following:

Prompt	You type	Meaning
Data file (.REC):	HEALTH	Name of data file to be created
Choose one:	2	Create new data file from .QES file
New questionnaire file (.QES):	HEALTH	Template to create data file from
OK:	Y	Everything is OK

Press **F4** to create the new data file (HEALTH.REC). The data entry screen appears.

Now enter some data into the HEALTH.REC file. When you have finished entering data press **F10** to quit.

Advanced analysis

A sample dataset is stored in the file ADVANCED.REC (you should have already copied this file over from your CD-ROM to the EPI6 directory – if you have not done this, refer to p. 46). Start ANALYSIS and open the file ADVANCED.REC by typing:

- READ ADVANCED.REC
- Press ⟨ENTER⟩

Note: if you have difficulties working with this file, it may be stored as a 'Read-Only' file. To correct this, please see instructions on p. 56.

Converting dates of birth into age values

At the EPI6> prompt type the following commands:

```
1 DEFINE AGE # # #
2 Press ⟨ENTER⟩
3 LET AGE = ("01/02/2003" – DOB) DIV 365.25
4 Press ⟨ENTER⟩
```

You have now created a numeric field called AGE and converted all of the dates of birth into age values in whole years and placed them in the AGE field. This will represent the ages of patients at 1 February 2003.

To examine the ages type:

- FREQ AGE
- Press ⟨ENTER⟩

Examine the output carefully (as shown below) and answer the questions that follow it.

```
AGE   | Freq  Percent   Cum.
------+----------------------
  23  |    1    2.0%     2.0%
  26  |    1    2.0%     4.0%
  27  |    2    4.0%     8.0%
  28  |    3    6.0%    14.0%
  29  |    1    2.0%    16.0%
  31  |    5   10.0%    26.0%
  32  |    2    4.0%    30.0%
  33  |    1    2.0%    32.0%
  34  |    2    4.0%    36.0%
  36  |    1    2.0%    38.0%
  39  |    3    6.0%    44.0%
  40  |    3    6.0%    50.0%
  41  |    4    8.0%    58.0%
  43  |    2    4.0%    62.0%
  44  |    2    4.0%    66.0%
  45  |    1    2.0%    68.0%
  46  |    1    2.0%    70.0%
  47  |    1    2.0%    72.0%
  49  |    1    2.0%    74.0%
  50  |    3    6.0%    80.0%
  51  |    2    4.0%    84.0%
  52  |    2    4.0%    88.0%
  54  |    2    4.0%    92.0%
  57  |    1    2.0%    94.0%
  58  |    1    2.0%    96.0%
  60  |    1    2.0%    98.0%
  70  |    1    2.0%   100.0%
------+----------------------
Total |   50  100.0%
```

	Total	Sum	Mean	Variance	Std Dev	Std Err
	50	2043	40.860	110.041	10.490	1.484

	Minimum	25%ile	Median	75%ile	Maximum	Mode
	23.000	31.000	40.500	50.000	70.000	31.000

Questions 1

1 How many ages are recorded?
2 What are the minimum and maximum ages?
3 What is the most common age?
4 How often is it recorded?
5 What is the standard deviation of the ages?
6 Is this group of ages homogeneous, and why?

Creating age bands

Type the following commands:

1 DEFINE AGEGROUP ⟨AAAAA⟩
2 Press ⟨ENTER⟩
3 RECODE AGE TO AGEGROUP 21–40 = "21–40" 41–60 = "41–60"
  61–80 = "61–80"
4 Press ⟨ENTER⟩

This recodes all of the age values into the age bands you have specified.
  To examine the age groups, type:

• FREQ AGEGROUP
• Press ⟨ENTER⟩

which produces the following output:

```
AGEGROUP |  Freq  Percent    Cum.
---------+-----------------------
21-40    |    25   50.0%      50.0%
41-60    |    24   48.0%      98.0%
61-80    |     1    2.0%     100.0%
---------+-----------------------
   Total |    50  100.0%
```

The ages are now grouped into age bands.

Converting height and weight fields into BMI values

Type the following commands:

1 DEFINE BMI # #
2 Press ⟨ENTER⟩
3 LET BMI = (WEIGHT/HEIGHT^2)
4 Press ⟨ENTER⟩

You have now created a new number field called BMI, converted all of the heights and weights into BMI values (rounded to the nearest whole number) and put them into the BMI field.
  To examine the BMI values, type:

• FREQ BMI
• Press ⟨ENTER⟩

Examine the output (you really only need to look at the statistics at the bottom):

```
BMI

        Total        Sum       Mean   Variance    Std Dev    Std Err
          50        1324     26.480     40.459      6.361      0.900

      Minimum     25%ile     Median     75%ile    Maximum       Mode
       16.000     22.000     27.000     29.000     43.000     25.000
```

Questions 2

1 What is the most common BMI value?
2 Is this a good measure of the central tendency of the distribution of BMI values?
3 What are the minimum and maximum BMI values?

The IF . . . . THEN command

We will now use the IF . . . THEN command to attach descriptions to the BMIs recorded, grouping the subjects into 'underweight', 'normal', 'overweight' or 'obese'.
   Type:

```
 1  DEFINE BMIGROUP ⟨AAAAAAAAAAAAAA⟩
 2  Press ⟨ENTER⟩
 3  IF BMI <19 THEN BMIGROUP = "UNDERWEIGHT"
 4  Press ⟨ENTER⟩
 5  IF BMI >=19 AND <=25 THEN BMIGROUP = "NORMAL"
 6  Press ⟨ENTER⟩
 7  IF BMI >25 AND <=30 THEN BMIGROUP = "OVERWEIGHT"
 8  Press ⟨ENTER⟩
 9  IF BMI >30 THEN BMIGROUP = "OBESE"
10  Press ⟨ENTER⟩
```

To examine the BMI groups, type:

• FREQ BMIGROUP
• Press ⟨ENTER⟩

Examine the output carefully (as shown below) and answer the questions.

BMIGROUP	Freq	Percent	Cum.
normal	14	28.0%	28.0%
obese	11	22.0%	50.0%
overweight	19	38.0%	88.0%
underweight	6	12.0%	100.0%
Total	50	100.0%	

Questions 3

1 What percentage of the subjects had 'normal' BMI values?
2 What percentage of the subjects were 'underweight'?
3 What percentage of the subjects were 'obese'?

Saving your analysis

You may wish to save all the commands you have used in this tutorial so they can be run again without you having to manually enter all of the commands again. To do so type:

* SAVE ADVANCED.PGM
* Press ⟨ENTER⟩

To run the analysis program again, type:

* RUN ADVANCED.PGM
* Press ⟨ENTER⟩

Calculating sample sizes

Use STATCALC to calculate the sample sizes for the following.

1 A population of 600; minimum standard 75%; confidence level of 90%
From the PROGRAMS menu:

1 Select STATCALC
2 Select SAMPLE SIZE & POWER
3 Select POPULATION SURVEY
4 Type the size of population – 600
5 Type 75 in EXPECTED FREQUENCY
6 Type 70 in WORST ACCEPTABLE RESULT (allow a possible 5% error for your minimum standard)

7 Press **F4**
8 Read off the sample size required for 90% confidence

2 *A population of 2500; minimum standard 90%; confidence level 99%*
From the PROGRAMS menu:

1 Select STATCALC
2 Select SAMPLE SIZE & POWER
3 Select POPULATION SURVEY
4 Type the size of population – 2500
5 Type 90 in EXPECTED FREQUENCY
6 Type 85 in WORST ACCEPTABLE RESULT (allow a possible 5% error
   for your minimum standard)
7 Press **F4**
8 Read off the sample size required for 99% confidence

Answers 1

1 50.
2 Minimum 23; maximum 70.
3 31.
4 Five times.
5 10.490.
6 No – there is a difference of 47 years between the highest and lowest
   ages and the ages are evenly spread throughout this range.

Answers 2

1 25 (the mode).
2 Yes, this value is reasonably similar to both the median and mean BMI
   values in this sample. There is a difference of 2.0 between the median
   and the mode, while the mean lies roughly in the middle.
3 Minimum 16; maximum 43.

Answers 3

1 28%.
2 12%.
3 22%.

Calculating sample sizes answers

Answer 1: 152.
Answer 2: 218.

10

Example audit protocols

To illustrate how Epi Info can effectively be used with clinical audit, we have included two example audit protocols. These are quite basic examples, but aim to illustrate how simple and useful both audit and Epi Info can be. The protocols are accompanied by ready-made Epi Info .QES and .REC files on the CD-ROM supplied with this book. Data have been entered into the .REC files, which you can analyse. You have the option of using the .QES files in their present form, or amending them to suit your own audit requirements. Full instructions for using the .QES files for your own audit can be found in Chapter 11.

Audit of diabetes in primary care

Aim

The aim of this audit is to ensure that all appropriate information is being recorded in patients' notes or computer records.

Criteria and standards

It is suggested that information should have been recorded for the following percentages of patients, although you may wish to set your own:

No.	Criteria	Standard %
1	**Foot examination** in past 18 months, if age >40	90
2	**Eye examination** in past 18 months, i.e. fundoscopy, by a trained professional, with pupils dilated with a mydriatic (at optometrist, hospital clinic or GP practice)	100 (unless registered blind)
3	**HbA1c** *or* **fasting blood glucose** measured in past 12 months	100
4	**Urine testing for microalbuminuria** in past 18 months, for patients with previously negative proteinuria test	100
5	**Cholesterol test** in past 24 months, if age >30	80
6	**BMI** measured in past 12 months	80
7	**Smoking status** recorded in last 5 years	80
8	**Blood pressure** checked in the past 12 months	80

Methodology

All patients with diagnosed diabetes should be identified either from the computer or from manual records. If you have a very large number of patients with diabetes, you may wish to randomly select a 30–50% sample, using a suitable random sampling technique.

These patients' records should then be examined and data entered onto the data collection sheet, summarising whether the above information has been recorded *within the specified period*.

Data analysis and results

The data will be analysed and results produced for each item of information.

Further discussion/change

Consideration should be given as to whether any changes should be implemented, and if so, what these should be. If indicated, these changes should be implemented immediately. The audit will be repeated after one year to establish whether the standards are still being achieved, and to assess the effectiveness of any changes.

A sample data collection form is shown opposite.

Audit of diabetes – data collection form

Sheet No. _____   Date _____

Enter the name (or identification) of each patient being studied, and complete each box as appropriate.
Refer to the accompanying sheet for instructions.

Enter a Y or a VALUE or a CODE (as indicated) if carried out/recorded. Enter an N if not carried out/recorded.
Enter N/A if the patient falls outside the criteria (e.g. in eye examination, if patient is blind).

Patient ID	Gender (M or F)	Age	NIDDM or IDDM (I or N)	Foot examination in past 18 months if age >40 (Y, N or N/A)	Eye examination in past 18 months (exc. Reg'd Blind) (Y or N or N/A)	HbA1c or fasting blood glucose in past 12 months (HbA1c value or N/A)	Urine test in past 18 months, for patients with −ve proteinuria test (Y, N or N/A)	Cholesterol test in past 24 months if age >30 (Y, N or N/A)	BMI measured in past 12 months (BMI value or N)	Smoking status in last 5 years (Y or N)	Blood pressure recorded in past 12 months (Y or N)	Systolic BP (mmHg)	Diastolic BP (mmHg)

Analysis of data using Epi Info

We will now carry out a basic analysis of this audit's data. You may wish to explore further on your own. Open Epi Info, and the ANALYSIS program. Then open the dataset called DIABETES.REC by typing:

• READ DIABETES

and pressing ⟨ENTER⟩.

The data fields used in this dataset are as follows:

Data field description	Format	Epi Info field name
Patient identifier	Any value (maximum 40 characters)	PATIENTID
Gender	F or M	GENDER
Age	###	AGE
Diabetes type (NIDDM or IDDM)	N or I	TYPE
Foot examination done?	Y or N or NA	FOOT
Eye examination done?	Y or N or NA	EYE
HbA1c test done?	Y or N	HB
HbA1c value	##.##	HBVALUE
Urine test done?	Y or N or NA	URINE
Cholesterol test done?	Y or N or NA	CHOL
BMI measured?	Y or N	BMI
BMI value	###	BMIVALUE
Smoking status recorded?	Y or N	SMOKING
Blood pressure recorded?	Y or N	BP
Systolic blood pressure (mmHg)	###	SYSTOLIC
Diastolic blood pressure (mmHg)	###	DIASTOLIC

You will see that data for 400 patients have been included. Before assessing how many of the audit standards have been met, we will start by looking at some basic characteristics of this practice population. First of all, let's take a look at the proportions of male and female patients. Type:

• FREQ GENDER

and press ⟨ENTER⟩.

The following frequency table will be produced:

```
GENDER |  Freq  Percent   Cum.
-------+----------------------
  F    |   191   47.8%    47.8%
  M    |   209   52.3%   100.0%
-------+----------------------
 Total |   400  100.0%
```

So we have a slight excess of males (52.3%). Alternatively, this can be dispayed as a pie chart. Type:

- PIE GENDER

and press ⟨ENTER⟩.

And the following chart will be produced:

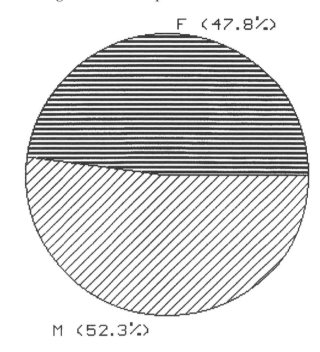

Next, we will look at the ages of this population. Type:

- FREQ AGE

and press ⟨ENTER⟩.

The resulting frequency table looks like this:

```
AGE  |  Freq  Percent    Cum.
------+----------------------
   8  |    1    0.3%     0.3%
  11  |    1    0.3%     0.5%
  17  |    1    0.3%     0.8%
  20  |    1    0.3%     1.0%
  23  |    1    0.3%     1.3%
  25  |    1    0.3%     1.5%
  27  |    2    0.5%     2.0%
  28  |    3    0.8%     2.8%
  29  |    2    0.5%     3.3%
  30  |    2    0.5%     3.8%
  31  |    2    0.5%     4.3%
  32  |    2    0.5%     4.8%
  33  |    1    0.3%     5.0%
  34  |    1    0.3%     5.3%
  35  |    5    1.3%     6.5%
  36  |    3    0.8%     7.3%
  37  |    2    0.5%     7.8%
  38  |    3    0.8%     8.5%
  39  |    2    0.5%     9.0%
  40  |    4    1.0%    10.0%
  41  |    3    0.8%    10.8%
  42  |    7    1.8%    12.5%
  43  |    9    2.3%    14.8%
  44  |    6    1.5%    16.3%
  45  |    4    1.0%    17.3%
  46  |    6    1.5%    18.8%
  47  |    5    1.3%    20.0%
  48  |    2    0.5%    20.5%
  49  |    4    1.0%    21.5%
  50  |    8    2.0%    23.5%
  51  |    1    0.3%    23.8%
  52  |    6    1.5%    25.3%
  53  |    8    2.0%    27.3%
  54  |    7    1.8%    29.0%
  55  |    7    1.8%    30.8%
  56  |    7    1.8%    32.5%
  57  |    7    1.8%    34.3%
  58  |    7    1.8%    36.0%
  59  |   13    3.3%    39.3%
  60  |    8    2.0%    41.3%
  61  |   12    3.0%    44.3%
  62  |   10    2.5%    46.8%
  63  |    8    2.0%    48.8%
  64  |    9    2.3%    51.0%
  65  |   17    4.3%    55.3%
  66  |   14    3.5%    58.8%
  67  |   10    2.5%    61.3%
  68  |   12    3.0%    64.3%
  69  |    7    1.8%    66.0%
  70  |   16    4.0%    70.0%
  71  |   15    3.8%    73.8%
  72  |   11    2.8%    76.5%
  73  |    7    1.8%    78.3%
  74  |   10    2.5%    80.8%
  75  |    9    2.3%    83.0%
  76  |   11    2.8%    85.8%
  77  |    9    2.3%    88.0%
  78  |   10    2.5%    90.5%
  79  |    3    0.8%    91.3%
  80  |    5    1.3%    92.5%
  81  |    3    0.8%    93.3%
  82  |    1    0.3%    93.5%
  83  |    6    1.5%    95.0%
  84  |    2    0.5%    95.5%
  85  |    4    1.0%    96.5%
  86  |    4    1.0%    97.5%
  87  |    3    0.8%    98.3%
  88  |    1    0.3%    98.5%
  89  |    3    0.8%    99.3%
  91  |    2    0.5%    99.8%
  92  |    1    0.3%   100.0%
------+----------------------
Total |  400  100.0%


        Total       Sum       Mean   Variance    Std Dev    Std Err
          400     24551     61.377    230.697     15.189      0.759

      Minimum    25%ile     Median     75%ile    Maximum       Mode
        8.000    52.000     64.000     72.000     92.000     65.000
```

Student's "t", testing whether mean differs from zero.
T statistic = 80.820, df = 399   p-value = 0.00000

You can see that the average age is 61.377, ranging from 8 to 92. The median age is 64.000, and the most frequently occuring age (the mode) is 65, being recorded 17 times in all. It is clear therefore that there are more old patients than young in our practice population. To display these data in a bar chart, type:

• BAR AGE

and press ⟨ENTER⟩.

The bar chart looks something like this:

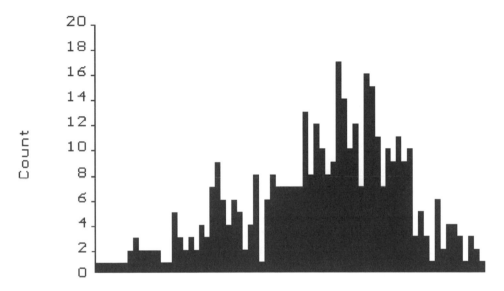

On your screen, you will also see some numbers crushed together along the bottom axis of the graph, though these are too close together to be readable.

We can now study the frequency of the two types of diabetes – non-insulin dependent diabetes (NIDDM) and insulin dependent diabetes (IDDM) – in these patients. By typing:

• FREQ TYPE

and pressing ⟨ENTER⟩.

It is apparent that 85.8% of the population had NIDDM (N) diabetes, while 14.3% had IDDM (I) diabetes.

TYPE	Freq	Percent	Cum.
I	57	14.3%	14.3%
N	343	85.8%	100.0%
Total	400	100.0%	

We will now examine the data to see whether the audit standards have been met. To see the result for **foot examinations**, type:

- FREQ FOOT

and press ⟨ENTER⟩.

You should see the following frequency table:

```
FOOT  | Freq  Percent   Cum.
------+----------------------
N     |   25    6.3%     6.3%
NA    |   34    8.5%    14.8%
Y     |  341   85.3%   100.0%
------+----------------------
Total |  400  100.0%
```

Although 85.3% of the patients received a foot examination according to the table, this figure is misleading, since 8.5% were not eligible for an examination (NA – presumably because they were aged 40 or less). What we really need is the percentage of eligible patients who received the examination. We can find this by selecting only the eligible patients. To do this, type:

1 SELECT FOOT="Y" OR FOOT="N"
2 Press ⟨ENTER⟩
3 FREQ FOOT
4 Press ⟨ENTER⟩

By selecting only the 'Y's and 'N's, we are excluding the patients who did not need a foot examination, according to the audit protocol ('NA's). The new frequency table looks like this:

```
Current selection: foot="Y" or foot="N"

FOOT  | Freq  Percent   Cum.
------+----------------------
N     |   25    6.8%     6.8%
Y     |  341   93.2%   100.0%
------+----------------------
Total |  366  100.0%
```

Now that the ineligible patients have been excluded, the true percentage of patients receiving a foot examination (in the past 18 months) according to the audit protocol has increased to 93.2%.

Type SELECT and press ⟨ENTER⟩ to clear the selection before moving on.

The next standard to check is **eye examinations**. Typing FREQ EYE and pressing ⟨ENTER⟩ produces the following frequency table:

```
EYE    |  Freq   Percent    Cum.
-------+----------------------------
N      |   117    29.3%     29.3%
Y      |   283    70.8%    100.0%
-------+----------------------------
Total  |   400   100.0%
```

Although the audit protocol excludes registered blind patients from this examination (obviously), none were recorded, so there are no 'NA's in the table. You can therefore see that 70.8% of patients received this examination in the past 18 months.

Standard number 3 is **HbA1c** (or **fasting blood glucose**) testing. Type FREQ HB and press ⟨ENTER⟩ to get the following table:

```
HB     |  Freq   Percent    Cum.
-------+----------------------------
N      |   107    26.8%     26.8%
Y      |   293    73.3%    100.0%
-------+----------------------------
Total  |   400   100.0%
```

This indicates that 73.3% of patients received an HbA1c or fasting blood glucose test within the past 12 months.

With the next standard (**urine testing**), typing FREQ URINE and pressing ⟨ENTER⟩ shows that 78.3% of patients (with previously negative proteinuria tests) received a urine test within the past 12 months:

```
URINE  |  Freq   Percent    Cum.
-------+----------------------------
N      |    87    21.8%     21.8%
Y      |   313    78.3%    100.0%
-------+----------------------------
Total  |   400   100.0%
```

Note that no 'NA's were recorded.

For standard number 5, cholesterol testing, typing FREQ CHOL and pressing ⟨ENTER⟩ reveals that 13 patients were not eligible for this test and therefore need to be excluded from the analysis of this standard.

```
CHOL   |  Freq   Percent    Cum.
-------+----------------------------
N      |   180    45.0%     45.0%
NA     |    13     3.3%     48.3%
Y      |   207    51.8%    100.0%
-------+----------------------------
Total  |   400   100.0%
```

This is done by using the SELECT command, in the same way as we did with the foot examination example earlier. To select only the eligible patients (who should be aged over 30, according to the protocol), type:

1 SELECT CHOL="Y" OR CHOL="N"
2 Press ⟨ENTER⟩
3 FREQ CHOL
4 Press ⟨ENTER⟩

```
        Current selection: CHOL="Y" OR CHOL="N"

        CHOL  |  Freq  Percent    Cum.
        ------+----------------------
        N     |   180   46.5%    46.5%
        Y     |   207   53.5%   100.0%
        ------+----------------------
        Total |   387  100.0%
```

So 53.5% of patients aged over 30 received a cholesterol test in the past 24 months.

You may now like to produce the remaining frequency tables for **BMI**, **smoking** and **blood pressure**. They should appear as follows:

```
        BMI   |  Freq  Percent    Cum.
        ------+----------------------
        N     |    58   14.5%    14.5%
        Y     |   342   85.5%   100.0%
        ------+----------------------
        Total |   400  100.0%
```

```
        SMOKING   |  Freq  Percent    Cum.
        ----------+----------------------
        N         |    30    7.5%     7.5%
        Y         |   370   92.5%   100.0%
        ----------+----------------------
            Total |   400  100.0%
```

```
        BP    |  Freq  Percent    Cum.
        ------+----------------------
        N     |    57   14.3%    14.3%
        Y     |   343   85.8%   100.0%
        ------+----------------------
        Total |   400  100.0%
```

You can now summarise the standards and the results we obtained in the table, below:

No.	Criteria	Standard %	Recorded %	Standard achieved?
1	**Foot examination** in past 18 months, if age > 40	90	93.2	Yes
2	**Eye examination** in past 18 months, i.e. fundoscopy, by a trained professional, with pupils dilated with a mydriatic (at optometrist, hospital clinic or GP practice)	100 (unless registered blind)	70.8	No
3	**HbA1c** *or* **fasting blood glucose** measured in past 12 months	100	73.3	No
4	**Urine testing for microalbuminuria** in past 18 months, for patients with previously negative proteinuria test	100	78.3	No
5	**Cholesterol test** in past 24 months, if age > 30	80	53.5	No
6	**BMI** measured in past 12 months	80	85.5	Yes
7	**Smoking status** recorded in last 5 years	80	92.5	Yes
8	**Blood pressure** checked in the past 12 months	80	85.8	Yes

This audit has therefore shown that standards for foot examinations plus recording of BMI, smoking status and blood pressure have been met. There were, however, quite substantial shortfalls in performance for eye examination, HbA1c, urine and cholesterol testing – all of these were between 20 and 30% below the minimum standard.

As well as using Epi Info to check whether the standards have been met, you could go further and see if there is any significant association between two categorical variables. For example, could it be that females are more likely than males to receive a blood pressure check? It is possible that more women will have this check because they are more likely to consult a GP for symptoms, or are better at complying with follow-up appointments. Or could there be some systematic tendency for health professionals to check womens' blood pressure more frequently than male patients? An examination of the data reveals that 170 out of 191 women (89%) have had their blood pressure checked, compared to 173 out of 209 men (82.8%). Although a difference exists, is this statistically significant or just a chance occurrence?

Because the data here are categorical (i.e. being *either* female *or* male, and *either* receiving *or* not receiving a blood pressure check) you can use the **chi-squared test** to test for significant association between these variables. The TABLES command is used, followed by two categorical variables. It is usual to type the variable relating to an exposure first, followed by the variable relating to an outcome. In this case, gender is the exposure and BP (blood pressure testing) is the outcome. This is because we are testing to see if being female is associated with receiving a blood pressure check – under these circumstances, receiving a blood pressure check cannot *result* in a patient being female, but it is possible that being female makes it more likely that a blood pressure check will be carried out.

To carry out this test, type:

* TABLES GENDER BP

and press ⟨ENTER⟩. The screen output appears below:

```
                      BP
     GENDER    |    N      Y    |  Total
     ----------+----------------+------
         F     |    21     170   |   191
         M     |    36     173   |   209
     ----------+----------------+------
        Total  |    57     343   |   400



                         Single Table Analysis

     Odds ratio                                          0.59
     Cornfield 95% confidence limits for OR              0.32 < OR <    1.10
     Maximum likelihood estimate of OR (MLE)             0.59
     Exact 95% confidence limits for MLE                 0.32 < OR <    1.09
     Exact 95% Mid-P limits for MLE                      0.33 < OR <    1.06
     Probability of MLE <=  0.59 if population OR = 1.0  0.05020098

     RISK RATIO(RR)(Outcome:BP=N; Exposure:GENDER=F)     0.64
     95% confidence limits for RR                        0.39 < RR <    1.05

                 Ignore risk ratio if case control study




                        Chi-Squares   P-values
                        -----------   --------

           Uncorrected:       3.17    0.07500122
           Mantel-Haenszel:   3.16    0.07536610
           Yates corrected:   2.68    0.10157285
```

For a chi-squared test, the information in the middle section of the box can be ignored.

The uncorrected p value is 0.07500122, and the Yates' corrected p value is 0.10157285. As these p values are *more than* 0.05 (the usual threshold of statistical significance), you can conclude that there is no significant association between being female and receiving a blood pressure check in this sample of patients.

You might like to experiment by doing chi-squared tests on other variables, such as TABLES GENDER CHOL (to see if there is any association between gender and receiving a cholesterol check) or TABLES TYPE EYE (to see if there is an association between diabetes type and receiving an eye check), for example.

You could also perform the **independent *t*-test**. This could, for example, be done to test whether there is a significant difference in mean HbA1c values between patients with NIDDM and IDDM type diabetes. The mean HbA1c value for patients with NIDDM diabetes is 6.878, compared to a mean of 7.300 for patients with IDDM diabetes. To test whether this difference is significant, type:

- MEANS HBVALUE TYPE

and press ⟨ENTER⟩.

An excerpt from your screen output is shown below:

```
TYPE            Obs        Total        Mean    Variance    Std Dev
I                34          248        7.300      5.940      2.437
N               198         1362        6.878      4.168      2.042
Difference                              0.422

TYPE          Minimum      25%ile      Median     75%ile    Maximum        Mode
I               4.000       5.500       7.000      8.800     14.600       5.800
N               3.200       5.200       6.700      8.300     15.700       5.200

                              ANOVA
                (For normally distributed data only)

Variation          SS    df          MS   F statistic    p-value    t-value
Between         5.173     1       5.173         1.170   0.280581   1.081560
Within       1017.102   230       4.422
Total        1022.275   231

               Bartlett's test for homogeneity of variance
     Bartlett's chi square =   1.908   deg freedom =  1   p-value = 0.167192

         The variances are homogeneous with 95% confidence.
     If samples are also normally distributed, ANOVA results can be used.


  Mann-Whitney or Wilcoxon Two-Sample Test (Kruskal-Wallis test for two groups)

  Kruskal-Wallis H (equivalent to Chi square) =      0.680
                        Degrees of freedom =           1
                               p value =       0.409676
```

The text beneath the ANOVA results indicates that the ANOVA results can be used. The p value is therefore 0.280581. As this is *more than* 0.05, we can conclude that there is no significant difference between HbA1c values between patients with NIDDM and IDDM types of diabetes.

Again, you can carry out other independent *t*-tests, by typing: MEANS AGE GENDER (to test whether the mean ages of males are significantly different from those of females) or MEANS BMIVALUE TYPE (to test whether the mean BMI values of patients with NIDDM are significantly different to those of patients with IDDM), for example.

Audit of angina management in primary care

Aims

This audit aims to assess the following areas of primary care angina management:

- identification and treatment of risk factors, and lifestyle advice given
- use of drug therapy.

The audit will help the practice to evaluate its angina management and highlight areas where patient care could be improved.

Criteria and standards

No.	Criteria	Standard %
1	Prescribe or advise low dose aspirin (75–150 mg/day), unless contraindicated	100
2	Patients should be given lifestyle advice on all of the following: smoking, weight reduction, exercise and alcohol intake	100
3	Identify and treat other coronary risk factors (e.g. hypertension, diabetes, hyperlipidaemia)	100
4	Prescribe a short acting nitrate (to use p.r.n. and prophylactically)	100
5	Prescribe a beta-blocker in the absence of contraindications	100

Methodology

Patient identification

Practices should first identify patients to be entered into the audit. These should be patients meeting *any* of the following criteria:

- Are known to have angina.
- Are known to have ischaemic heart disease (IHD).
- Are receiving repeat prescriptions for short-acting nitrates.

A list of these patients should be produced, including age, gender and ethnic group if possible. Practices may wish to use identification numbers instead of names. If a large number of patients is identified, you may wish to randomly select a 10% sample using a suitable random sampling technique.

Data collection

The notes of each selected patient should then be examined and data entered onto the data collection form. This records the following details:

- patient ID
- age
- sex
- ethnic group
- low-dose aspirin prescribed (unless contraindicated or advised to take)?
- smoking advice given?
- weight reduction advice given?
- exercise advice given?
- alcohol advice given?
- BP recorded in <12 months?
- blood glucose test in <12 months?
- cholesterol tested in <12 months?
- short-acting nitrate prescribed?
- beta-blocker prescribed (unless contraindicated)?

Data analysis

All data will be held in strict confidence.

Further discussion/change

Using the results obtained, the practice team should consider whether performance has met the standards originally set, and what further action would be appropriate to meet them in the future. The audit will be repeated after one year to establish whether the standards are still being achieved, and to assess the effectiveness of any changes.

A sample data collection form is shown overleaf.

Audit of angina management in primary care – data collection form

Sheet No. _____   Date _____

(Key: **Y** = Yes, **N** = No, **X** = contraindicated, **Z** = n/a)

(Ethnic group key: **W** = White UK, **WO** = White other, **R** = Irish, **V** = Vietnamese, **I** = Indian; **P** = Pakistani, **B** = Bangladeshi, **C** = Chinese, **BA** = Black African, **BC** = Black Caribbean, **BO** = Black other, **O** = Other)

Patient ID	Age	Sex (M/F)	Ethnic group (see list above)	Aspirin prescribed or advised (Y/N/X)	Smoking advice (Y/N)	Weight advice (Y/N)	Exercise advice (Y/N)	Alcohol advice (Y/N)	BP record <12 months (Y/N)	Blood glucose <12 months (Y/N)	Cholesterol <12 months (Y/N)	Short-acting nitrate (Y/N/X/Z)	Beta-blocker (Y/N/X/Z)

Analysis of data using Epi Info

We will now carry out a basic analysis of the angina audit's data. As with the previous audit, you may also wish to explore further on your own. Open Epi Info, and the ANALYSIS program. Then open the dataset called ANGINA.REC by typing:

- READ ANGINA

and pressing ⟨ENTER⟩.
    The data fields used in this dataset are as follows:

Data field description	Format	Epi Info field name
Patient identifier	Any value (maximum 10 characters)	PATIENTID
Age	# #	AGE
Sex	F or M	SEX
Ethnic Group	W/WO/R/V/I/P/B/C/BA/ BC/BO/O (see key on data collection form)	ETHNIC
Aspirin prescribed or advised?	Y or N or X	ASPIRIN
Smoking advice given?	Y or N	SMOKING
Weight advice given?	Y or N	WEIGHT
Exercise advice given?	Y or N	EXERCISE
Alcohol advice given?	Y or N	ALCOHOL
Blood pressure recorded?	Y or N	BP
Blood glucose recorded?	Y or N	BLOOD
Cholesterol recorded?	Y or N	CHOL
Short-acting nitrate prescribed?	Y or N or X or Z	NITRATE
Beta-blocker prescribed?	Y or N or X or Z	BETA

You may notice a couple of differences to the earlier diabetes fields – the word 'sex' is used instead of 'gender', and the age field has only two characters (adequate for many audits, though only allows ages of up to 99).
    You will see that data for 300 patients with angina have been included. Before assessing how many of the audit standards have been met, let's again start by looking at some basic characteristics of this practice population. You can begin with a look at the ages of this population. Type:

- FREQ AGE

and press ⟨ENTER⟩.

The statistics summary in the frequency table looks like this:

Total	Sum	Mean	Variance	Std Dev	Std Err
300	20241	67.470	139.768	11.822	0.683

Minimum	25%ile	Median	75%ile	Maximum	Mode
25.000	59.000	68.000	77.000	97.000	70.000

The list of ages, frequencies, percentages, etc., has been omitted here. You can see, however, that the mean age is 67.470, and that ages range from 25 to 97.

Next, you can examine the proportions of male and female patients. Type:

• FREQ SEX

and press ⟨ENTER⟩.

The following frequency table will be produced:

SEX	Freq	Percent	Cum.
F	133	44.3%	44.3%
M	167	55.7%	100.0%
Total	300	100.0%	

There is an excess of male patients (55.7%).

Next, you might like to examine the frequencies of ethnic group. To do this, type:

• FREQ ETHNIC

and press ⟨ENTER⟩.

For clarity, the names of the ethnic groups have been added alongside the audit codes.

	ETHNIC	Freq	Percent	Cum.
Bangladeshi	B	7	2.3%	2.3%
Black Caribbean	BC	11	3.7%	6.0%
Chinese	C	3	1.0%	7.0%
Indian	I	43	14.3%	21.3%
Pakistani	P	7	2.3%	23.7%
Irish	R	3	1.0%	24.7%
White UK	W	225	75.0%	99.7%
White Other	WO	1	0.3%	100.0%
	Total	300	100.0%	

So the majority of these patients with angina are 'White UK' (75.0%), followed by 'Indian' (14.3%) and 'Black Caribbean' (3.7%). The *least* frequently recorded ethnic group is 'White other' (0.3%).

Now that the basic population characteristics have been covered, you can continue by determining whether the audit standards have been met.

The first standard is aspirin. Typing FREQ ASPIRIN and pressing ⟨ENTER⟩ reveals that 28 patients have not received aspirin, due to contraindications (**X** – see key on data collection form):

```
ASPIRIN |  Freq  Percent   Cum.
--------+----------------------
N       |    96   32.0%    32.0%
X       |    28    9.3%    41.3%
Y       |   176   58.7%   100.0%
--------+----------------------
  Total |   300  100.0%
```

To eliminate these 28 patients from the analysis, type the following:

1 SELECT ASPIRIN = "Y" OR ASPIRIN = "N"
2 Press ⟨ENTER⟩
3 FREQ ASPIRIN
4 Press ⟨ENTER⟩

The frequency table now looks like this:

```
    Current selection: aspirin="Y" or aspirin="N"

ASPIRIN |  Freq  Percent   Cum.
--------+----------------------
N       |    96   35.3%    35.3%
Y       |   176   64.7%   100.0%
--------+----------------------
  Total |   272  100.0%
```

So after the patients for whom aspirin is contraindicated have been eliminated, the true proportion of patients receiving aspirin is 64.7%.

Type SELECT and press ⟨ENTER⟩ to clear the selection before moving on.

You might now like to produce frequency tables for the other standards. The results are as follows:

- Smoking advice – 83.3%
- Weight advice – 75.3%
- Exercise advice – 65.0%
- Alcohol advice – 75.3%
- Blood pressure recorded – 77.3%
- Blood glucose recorded – 33.3%
- Cholesterol recorded – 40.0%
- Short-acting nitrate prescribed – 61.7% (after excluding two contraindications [X])
- Beta-blocker prescribed – 56.9% (after excluding 31 contraindications [X] and 2 N/As [Z])

You can now summarise the standards and these results in the table, below:

No.	Criteria	Standard %	Recorded %	Standard achieved?
1	Prescribe or advise low dose aspirin (75–150 mg/day), unless contraindicated	100	64.7	No
2	Patients should be given lifestyle advice on all of the following:			
	– smoking	100	83.3	No
	– weight reduction	100	75.3	No
	– exercise	100	65.0	No
	– alcohol intake	100	75.3	No
3	Identify and treat other coronary risk factors			
	– hypertension (blood pressure [BP] field)	100	77.3	No
	– diabetes (blood glucose [BLOOD] field)	100	33.3	No
	– hyperlipidaemia (cholesterol [CHOL] field)	100	40.0	No
4	Prescribe a short-acting nitrate (to use p.r.n. and prophylactically)	100	61.7	No
5	Prescribe a beta-blocker in the absence of contraindications	100	56.9	No

It is clear that none of the audit standards has been met. The results for blood glucose and cholesterol testing are especially disappointing.

You can now consider whether any further analysis, including statistical tests, should be performed. For example, could there be a systematic tendency for males to receive aspirin, rather than females? In this case, the chi-squared test can be used to test for association between sex and receiving aspirin.

To carry out this test, type:

1 SELECT ASPIRIN = "Y" OR ASPIRIN = "N"
   (to eliminate contraindicated patients from the analysis)
2 Press ⟨ENTER⟩
3 TABLES SEX ASPIRIN
4 Press ⟨ENTER⟩

Your screen output will look like this:

```
Current selection: aspirin="Y" or aspirin="N"

                        ASPIRIN
SEX           |     N      Y | Total
----------+-----------------+------
        F |    41     77 |   118
        M |    55     99 |   154
----------+-----------------+------
    Total |    96    176 |   272


                  Single Table Analysis

Odds ratio                                          0.96
Cornfield 95% confidence limits for OR              0.56 < OR <    1.64
Maximum likelihood estimate of OR (MLE)             0.96
Exact 95% confidence limits for MLE                 0.56 < OR <    1.63
Exact 95% Mid-P limits for MLE                      0.58 < OR <    1.59
Probability of MLE <=  0.96 if population OR = 1.0   0.48565646

RISK RATIO(RR)(Outcome:ASPIRIN=N; Exposure:SEX=F)   0.97
95% confidence limits for RR                        0.70 < RR <    1.35

            Ignore risk ratio if case control study



                      Chi-Squares   P-values
                      -----------   --------

          Uncorrected:      0.03    0.86842868
     Mantel-Haenszel:       0.03    0.86866857
     Yates corrected:       0.00    0.96996770
```

The uncorrected and Yates' corrected p values are *more than* 0.05, indicating that there is no significant association.

Type SELECT and press ⟨ENTER⟩ to clear the selection before moving on.

Could there be an association between other factors, however? To explore association between sex and receiving a beta-blocker, type:

1 SELECT BETA = "Y" OR BETA = "N"
   (to eliminate contraindicated and N/A patients from the analysis)
2 Press ⟨ENTER⟩
3 TABLES SEX BETA
4 Press ⟨ENTER⟩

Your screen output will look like this:

```
Current selection: beta="Y" or beta="N"

                          BETA
SEX           |      N      Y | Total
--------------+---------------+------
           F  |     59     57 |  116
           M  |     56     95 |  151
--------------+---------------+------
       Total  |    115    152 |  267


                    Single Table Analysis

Odds ratio                                         1.76
Cornfield 95% confidence limits for OR             1.04 < OR <    2.97
Maximum likelihood estimate of OR (MLE)            1.75
Exact 95% confidence limits for MLE                1.04 < OR <    2.96
Exact 95% Mid-P limits for MLE                     1.07 < OR <    2.88
Probability of MLE >=  1.75 if population OR = 1.0  0.01664148

RISK RATIO(RR)(Outcome:BETA=N; Exposure:SEX=F)     1.37
95% confidence limits for RR                       1.04 < RR <    1.80

          Ignore risk ratio if case control study


                    Chi-Squares    P-values
                    -----------    --------

         Uncorrected:     5.08     0.02423836 <---
      Mantel-Haenszel:    5.06     0.02450574 <---
       Yates corrected:   4.53     0.03328210 <---
```

In total, 57 out of 116 females received a beta-blocker (49.1%), compared to 95 out of 151 men (62.9%). The uncorrected and Yates' corrected p values are *less than* 0.05, so there is a significant association between being male and receiving a beta-blocker.

As always, type SELECT and press ⟨ENTER⟩ to clear the selection before moving on.

In addition to chi-squared tests, you could carry out an independent *t*-test to explore whether there is a difference between the mean age of patients receiving various interventions. For example, could there be a significant difference in the mean ages of patients who have received and have not received a cholesterol check? (In other words, might there be a systematic tendency for older or younger patients to receive the check?) This can be tested by typing:

- MEANS AGE CHOL

and pressing ⟨ENTER⟩.

An excerpt from your screen output is shown below:

```
CHOL              Obs      Total      Mean    Variance    Std Dev
+                 120       7625     63.542    107.645     10.375
-                 180      12616     70.089    144.662     12.028
Difference                          -6.547

CHOL           Minimum     25%ile    Median     75%ile    Maximum      Mode
+               33.000     56.500    63.000     71.000     87.000    59.000
-               25.000     62.000    71.000     79.000     97.000    70.000

                                  ANOVA
                   (For normally distributed data only)

Variation           SS     df         MS   F statistic     p-value    t-value
Between       3086.361      1    3086.361       23.763    0.000002   4.874740
Within       38704.369    298     129.880
Total        41790.730    299


Bartlett's test for homogeneity of variance
    Bartlett's chi square =   3.040   deg freedom =   1    p-value = 0.081237

            The variances are homogeneous with 95% confidence.
    If samples are also normally distributed, ANOVA results can be used.


 Mann-Whitney or Wilcoxon Two-Sample Test (Kruskal-Wallis test for two groups)

 Kruskal-Wallis H (equivalent to Chi square) =      23.590
                      Degrees of freedom =           1
                              p value =         0.000001
```

The text beneath the ANOVA results indicates that the ANOVA results can be used. The p value is therefore 0.000002. As this is *less than* 0.05 (very much less!), there is a significant difference between the mean ages of patients who receive and do not receive a cholesterol check.

Similar tests could be carried out using:

- MEANS AGE BETA (p value = 0.007659 – significant)
- MEANS AGE BLOOD (p value = 0.059250 – not significant)

For MEANS AGE WEIGHT a significant p value is shown, but Epi Info uses a different test (due to the fact that the variances of the means are significantly different). You do not need to worry about how this is done, but it is always important to read the output and follow its instructions.

```
WEIGHT           Obs       Total       Mean   Variance   Std Dev
+                226       15039     66.544    119.814    10.946
-                 74        5202     70.297    192.431    13.872
Difference                           -3.753

WEIGHT        Minimum     25%ile     Median     75%ile    Maximum         Mode
+              25.000     60.000     67.000     75.000     89.000       70.000
-              37.000     59.000     70.000     80.000     97.000       66.000

                                     ANOVA
                    (For normally distributed data only)

Variation          SS   df           MS  F statistic    p-value     t-value
Between        785.213    1      785.213        5.706   0.017525    2.388805
Within       41005.517  298      137.602
Total        41790.730  299

              Bartlett's test for homogeneity of variance
      Bartlett's chi square =    6.632  deg freedom = 1   p-value = 0.010014

         Bartlett's Test shows the variances in the samples to differ.
            Use non-parametric results below rather than ANOVA.


  Mann-Whitney or Wilcoxon Two-Sample Test (Kruskal-Wallis test for two groups)

  Kruskal-Wallis H (equivalent to Chi square) =       4.132
                    Degrees of freedom =                   1
                            p value =          0.042078
```

In this case, you are directed to the non-parametric 'Kruskal-Wallis H' test result. This shows a p value of 0.042078, indicating a significant difference between the mean ages of patients who receive and do not receive weight reduction advice.

This practice therefore needs to take urgent action to ensure that all of its angina patients receive the appropriate interventions, and also consider taking steps to ensure that patients in all age groups are treated equally well.

11

Using an audit protocol as a template for your own audit

Each .QES file is a fully constructed data collection template, which you can either use in its present form, or customise to suit your requirements. To do this:

1 Access EPED, from the PROGRAMS menu.
2 Press **F2**, and select 'Open file this window', then press ⟨ENTER⟩.
3 If you have already copied the sample files over to your hard drive (as described on p. 46, type C:\EPI6\(filename).QES (e.g. C:\DIABETES.QES) *or* C:*.QES and press ⟨ENTER⟩ to see a listing of all the .QES files available. Use the arrow keys to select the file you want. If you have not copied the files over, insert the CD-ROM, and type D:\(filename).QES (e.g. D:\DIABETES.QES) *or* D:*.QES to see a listing of all the .QES files on the CD-ROM. Use the arrow keys to select the file you want.
4 Press ⟨ENTER⟩ and the file will open.
5 Customise the file by changing, adding or removing sections as desired or use the file in its original form if you are happy that it fits your needs.
6 Press **F2** and choose 'Save file to . . .'.
7 Type the destination drive (usually either A: if you are saving to a floppy disk or C: if you are saving it on your hard drive), followed by a

file name of up to eight characters ending in .QES. This filename should be different to the original one (e.g. C:\WAITING.QES) in order to avoid confusion or overwriting the original file. Then press ⟨ENTER⟩ to save the new file.

8 Press **F10** to exit the EPED program.
9 Select ENTER.
10 Type in the filename of your new .QES file (e.g. DIABET2.QES) and press ⟨ENTER⟩.
11 Type **2** (Create new data file from .QES file) and press ⟨ENTER⟩.
12 Type in the filename of your new .QES file (e.g. DIABET2.QES) and press ⟨ENTER⟩ *twice*.

A new entry file will now have been created. It will have the same filename as your QES file but will end in REC, denoting that it is a record file.

You can start entering data immediately, or exit out of ENTER by pressing **F10**.

Note: if you have difficulties working with the files, they may be stored as 'Read-Only' files. To correct this, please see instructions on p. 56.

References

- Antiplatelet Trialists' Collaboration (1994) Collaborative overview of randomised trials of antiplatelet therapy. Prevention of death, myocardial infarction, and stroke by prolonged antiplatelet therapy in various categories of patients. *BMJ.* **308**: 81–106.
- Armitage P and Berry G (2002) *Statistical Methods in Medical Research* (4e). Blackwell, Oxford.
- Berwick DM (1996) A primer on leading the improvement of systems. *BMJ.* **312**: 619–622.
- Bland M (1996) *Introduction to Medical Statistics* (2e). Oxford University Press, Oxford.
- Central Office for Research Ethics Committees (2003) When to apply for ethical review. On-line at: http://www.corec.org.uk/whenToApply.htm (accessed 26 Jan 2003).
- Chambers R and Boath E (2000) *Clinical Effectiveness and Clinical Governance Made Easy* (2e). Radcliffe Medical Press, Oxford.
- Dean AG, Dean JA, Coulombier D, Brendel KA, Smith DC, Burton AH, Dicker RC, Sullivan K, Fagan RF and Arner TG (1995) Epi Info, version 6: a word-processing, database and statistics program for public health on IBM-compatible microcomputers. Center for Disease Control and Prevention, Atlanta, Georgia, USA. (This program is free, and can be downloaded from the Internet: http://www.cdc.gov/epiinfo/ei6dnjp.htm.)
- Department of Health (1998) *A First Class Service: quality in the new NHS.* HMSO, London.
- Department of Health (2000) *National Service Framework for Coronary Heart Disease.* Department of Health, London (available on-line at: http://www.nelh.nhs.uk/nsf/chd/nsf/main/mainreport.htm).
- Donabedian A (1966) Evaluating the quality of medical care. *Millbank Memorial Fund Quarterly.* **44**: 166–204.
- Donaldson RJ and Donaldson LJ (2000) *Essential Public Health* (2e). Petroc Press, Newbury, Berks.
- Garside P (1998) Organisational context for quality: lessons from the fields of

organisational development and change management. *Quality in Health Care.* **7**(Suppl.): S8–S15.

- Kotter JP and Schlesinger LA (1979) Choosing strategies for change. *Harvard Business Review.* **57**(2): 106–14.
- Langley GJ, Nolan KM and Nolan TW (1992) *The Foundation of Improvement.* API Publishing, Silver Spring, MD.
- Lewin K (1951) *Field Theory in Social Science: selected theoretical papers* (D Cartwright, ed.). Harper Torchbooks, New York.
- National Institute for Clinical Excellence (2002) *Principles for Best Practice in Clinical Audit.* Radcliffe Medical Press, Oxford.
- National Institute for Clinical Excellence (2003) *About Clinical Audit.* NICE, London (available on-line at: www.nice.org.uk/cat.asp?c=164; accessed 26 Jan 2003).
- NHS Centre for Reviews and Dissemination (1999) Getting evidence into practice. *Effective Health Care Bulletin.* **5**(1): 11. NHS Centre for Reviews and Dissemination, University of York (available on-line at: http://www1.york.ac.uk/inst/crd/ehcb.htm).
- NHS Executive (1996) *Promoting Clinical Effectiveness.* NHS Executive, Leeds.
- Stewart A (2002) *Basic Statistics and Epidemiology: a practical guide.* Radcliffe Medical Press, Oxford.
- Upton T and Brooks B (1995) *Managing Change in the NHS.* Kogan Page, London.
- van Zwanenberg T and Harrison J (eds) (2000) *Clinical Governance in Primary Care.* Radcliffe Medical Press, Oxford.

Bibliography

- Abramson JH (1994) *Making Sense of Data: a self instructional manual on the interpretation of epidemiological data* (2e). Oxford University Press, Oxford.
- Altman DG (1991) *Practical Statistics for Medical Research*. Chapman & Hall, London.
- Armitage P and Berry G (2001) *Statistical Methods in Medical Research* (4e). Blackwell, Oxford.
- Baker R, Hearnshaw H and Robertson N (eds) (1998) *Implementing Change in Clinical Audit*. Wiley, Chichester.
- Bernard S (1998) *Clinical Audit in Physiotherapy*. Butterworth Heinemann, Oxford.
- Bland M (2000) *Introduction to Medical Statistics* (3e). Oxford University Press, Oxford.
- Bowers D (1996) *Statistics From Scratch: an introduction for health care professionals*. Wiley, Chichester.
- Bowers D (1997) *Statistics Further From Scratch: for health care professionals*. Wiley, Chichester.
- British Medical Association (1996) *Guidance Notes for the Commissioning of Clinical Audit*. BMA Professional Division Publications, London.
- Campbell MJ and Machin D (1999) *Medical Statistics: a commonsense approach* (3e). Wiley, Chichester.
- Chambers R and Boath E (2000) *Clinical Effectiveness and Clinical Governance Made Easy* (2e). Radcliffe Medical Press, Oxford.
- Chambers R and Wakely G (2000) *Making Clinical Governance Work For You*. Radcliffe Medical Press, Oxford.
- Commission for Health Improvement (2001) *A Guide to Clinical Governance Reviews in NHS Acute Trusts*. The Stationery Office, London.
- Dewar S (1999) *Clinical Governance Under Construction*. King's Fund, London.
- Diamond I and Jefferies J (2001) *Beginning Statistics: an introduction for social sciences*. Sage, London.
- Firth-Cozens J (1999) *Clinical Governance Development Needs in Health Service*

Staff. University of Northumbria at Newcastle, Faculty of Health, Social Work and Education, Newcastle.

- Godwin R (ed.) (1996) *Clinical Audit in Radiology.* Royal College of Radiologists, London.
- Higginson I (ed.) (1993) *Clinical Audit in Palliative Care.* Radcliffe Medical Press, Oxford.
- Iqbal Z, Chambers R and Woodmansey P (2001) *Implementing the National Service Framework for Coronary Heart Disease in Primary Care.* Radcliffe Medical Press, Oxford.
- Kinn S and Siann T (1993) *Computers and Clinical Audit.* Arnold, London.
- Kirkwood B (1988) *Essentials of Medical Statistics.* Blackwell, Oxford.
- Kogan M, Redfern S, Kober A, Norman I, Packwood T and Robinson S (1995) *Making Use of Clinical Audit.* Open University Press, Milton Keynes.
- Lilley R (1999) *Making Sense of Clinical Governance.* Radcliffe Medical Press, Oxford.
- Lim JNW and Burton T (2000) *What Elements Should Be Covered in a Clinical Governance Development Plan?* Nuffield Institute for Health, Oxford.
- Lim JNW, Harrison S and Brian A (2001) *Clinical Governance.* Nuffield Institute for Health, Oxford.
- Lugon M (1999) *Clinical Governance: making it happen.* Royal Society of Medicine Press, London.
- Lugon M and Secker Walker J (eds) (2001) *Advancing Clinical Governance.* Royal Society of Medicine Press, London.
- Mathers N, Williams M and Hancock B (eds) (2000) *Statistical Analysis in Primary Care.* Radcliffe Medical Press, Oxford.
- McSherry R and Pearce P (2001) *Clinical Governance.* Blackwell Science, Oxford.
- Miles A and Hill A (eds) (2001) *Clinical Governance and the NHS Reforms.* Aesculapius Medical Press, London.
- Morell C and Harvey G (1999) *The Clinical Audit Handbook.* Ballière Tindall, London.
- National Institute for Clinical Excellence (2002) *Principles for Best Practice in Clinical Audit.* Radcliffe Medical Press, Oxford.
- Patrick M and Davenhill R (eds) (1998) *Rethinking Clinical Audit.* Routledge, London.
- Po ALW (1998) *Dictionary of Evidence Based Medicine.* Radcliffe Medical Press, Oxford.
- Riordan J and Mockler D (1997) *Clinical Audit in Mental Health.* Wiley, Chichester.
- Rotherham G and Martin D (1999) *Clinical Governance in Primary Care.* NHS Confederation, London.
- Rowntree D (1981) *Statistics Without Tears: a primer for non-mathematicians.* Penguin, Harmondworth.
- Royal College of Radiologists (2000) *Clinical Governance and Revalidation.* Royal College of Radiologists, London.

- Sackett DL, Straus SE, Richardson WS, Rosenberg W and Haynes RB (2000) *Evidence-based Medicine: how to practice and teach EBM*. Churchill Livingston, Edinburgh.
- Samuel O, Grant J and Irvine D (eds) (1994) *Quality and Audit in General Practice – meanings and definitions*. Royal College of General Practitioners, London.
- Scotland AP (2000) *Clinical Governance: one year on*. Quay Books, Salisbury, Wilts.
- Simpson L and Robinson P (eds) (2002) *e-Clinical Governance: a guide for primary care*. Radcliffe Medical Press, Oxford.
- Stewart A (2002) *Basic Statistics and Epidemiology: a practical guide*. Radcliffe Medical Press, Oxford.
- Swage T (2000) *Clinical Governance in Healthcare Practice*. Butterworth Heinemann, Oxford.
- Swinscow TDV and Campbell MJ (2002) *Statistics at Square One* (10e). BMJ Publishing, London.
- van Zwanenberg T and Harrison J (2001) *Clinical Governance in Primary Care*. Radcliffe Medical Press, Oxford.
- Waine C (1994) *Clinical Audit*. Martin Dunitz, London.
- Walshe K (ed.) (1995) *Evaluating Clinical Audit*. Royal Society of Medicine Press, London.
- Walshe K and Spurgeon P (1997) *Clinical Audit Assessment Framework*. University of Birmingham, Birmingham.
- Walshe K, Walsh N, Schofield T and Blakeway-Philips C (eds) (1999) *Accreditation in Primary Care: towards clinical governance*. Radcliffe Medical Press, Oxford.
- Wilson J and Tingle J (1997) *Clinical Risk Management Modification: a route to clinical governance*. Butterworth Heinemann, Oxford.

Summary of Epi Info function keys

EPED

F1	Help
F2	File commands
F3	EPIAID – EPED tutorial
F4	Text commands
F5	Print
F6	Set-up codes
F7	Find/Move commands
F8	Block commands
F9	Save
F10	Done – exit from program

ENTER

⟨**Ctrl-N**⟩	New record
⟨**Ctrl-F**⟩	Search mode
F5	Print
F6	Delete record
F7	Browse – last record
F8	Browse – next record
F9	Choices (if legal values are set up)
F10	Done – exit from program

ENTER (search mode)

F2	Record number
F3	First record
F4	Next record
SF4	Previous record
F7	Browse – last record
F8	Browse – next record
⟨**Ctrl-N**⟩	New record

CHECK

	F1/F2	Min/Max range			
	F3	Repeat			
	F4	Must enter			
	F5	Link fields			
Legal	**F6**	Add	Shift-F6 Display	Ctrl-F6 Delete
Jump	**F7**	Add	Shift-F7 Display	Ctrl-F7 Delete
Codes	**F8**	Add	Shift-F8 Display	Ctrl-F8 Delete
	F9	Edit field			
	F10	Quit – exit program			

ANALYSIS

F1	Help
F2	Commands
F3	Variables
F4	Browse
F5	Printer on
F9	DOS
F10	Quit – exit program

Index